PUBLIC HEALTH IN THE 21ST CENTURY

INFLUENZA PANDEMIC: RESPONSE AND VACCINE CHALLENGES

PUBLIC HEALTH IN THE 21ST CENTURY

Additional books in this series can be found on Nova's website under the Series tab.

Additional E-books in this series can be found on Nova's website under the E-books tab.

PUBLIC HEALTH IN THE 21ST CENTURY

INFLUENZA PANDEMIC: RESPONSE AND VACCINE CHALLENGES

ADRIAN J. BUCKMAN
EDITOR

Nova Science Publishers, Inc.
New York

For permission to use material from this book please contact us:
Telephone 631-231-7269; Fax 631-231-8175
Web Site: http://www.novapublishers.com

NOTICE TO THE READER

Additional color graphics may be available in the e-book version of this book.

LIBRARY OF CONGRESS CATALOGING-IN-PUBLICATION DATA

Influenza pandemic : response and vaccine challenges / editor, Adrian J. Buckman.
p. ; cm.
"CRS Report for Congress"
Includes bibliographical references and index.
ISBN 978-1-61209-319-2 (hardcover)
1. Influenza--Government policy--United States. 2. Influenza vaccines--Government policy--United States. I. Buckman, Adrian J., editor.
[DNLM: 1. Influenza A Virus, H1N1 Subtype--United States. 2. Influenza, Human--United States. 3. Disease Outbreaks--United States. 4. Influenza Vaccines--United States. 5. Public Policy--United States. WC 515]
RA644.I6I534 2011
614.5'18--dc22
2010048355

Published by Nova Science Publishers, Inc. † New York

CONTENTS

Preface

On June 11th, 2009, in response to the global spread of a new strain of H1N1 influenza, the World Health Organization (WHO) declared the outbreak to be an influenza pandemic, the first since 1968. When the outbreak began, U.S. official adopted a response posture under the overall coordination of the Secretary of Homeland Security. This new book provides a synopsis of key events in the H1N1 pandemic response, followed by information about selected federal emergency management authorities and actions taken by DHS, HHS, and state and local authorities.

Chapter 1- On June 11, 2009, in response to the global spread of a new strain of H1N1 influenza ("flu"), the World Health Organization (WHO) declared the outbreak to be an influenza pandemic, the first since 1968. The novel "H1N1 swine flu" was first identified in California in late April. Since then, cases have been reported around the world.

When the outbreak began, U.S. officials adopted a response posture under the overall coordination of the Secretary of Homeland Security. Among other things, officials established a government-wide informational website (http://www.flu.gov), released antiviral drugs from the national stockpile, developed new diagnostic tests for the H1N1 virus, and published guidance for the clinical management of patients and the management of community and school outbreaks.

Chapter 2- Between April 2009 and February 2010, the United States experienced its most recent outbreak of pandemic influenza, this one resulting from the appearance of a novel strain ofType A, H1N1 virus. From the earliest recognition of the pandemic, public health officials in the United States moved rapidly to respond, but their efforts were impeded by unanticipated delays that arose in manufacturing what was supposed to be the most powerful tool for preventing widespread morbidity and mortality: a vaccine designed to protect against the 2009 H1N1 virus. Fortunately, the pathogenic potential of the 2009 H1N1 virus remained relatively mild, limiting morbidity and mortality, although a disproportionate number of deaths occurred among children and young ad ults. This less-than-optimal experience—one that developed despite the appropriate and energetic response of vaccine manufacturers and public health officials—raised new awareness of the limitations of the system by which influenza vaccines are produced today.

In: Influenza Pandemic: Response and Vaccine... ISBN: 978-1-61209-319-2
Editors: Adrian J. Buckman

Chapter 1

THE 2009 INFLUENZA PANDEMIC: AN OVERVIEW*

Sarah A. Lister and C. Stephen Redhead

SUMMARY

On June 11, 2009, in response to the global spread of a new strain of H1N1 influenza ("flu"), the World Health Organization (WHO) declared the outbreak to be an influenza pandemic, the first since 1968. The novel "H1N1 swine flu" was first identified in California in late April. Since then, cases have been reported around the world.

When the outbreak began, U.S. officials adopted a response posture under the overall coordination of the Secretary of Homeland Security. Among other things, officials established a government-wide informational website (http://www.flu.gov), released antiviral drugs from the national stockpile, developed new diagnostic tests for the H1N1 virus, and published guidance for the clinical management of patients and the management of community and school outbreaks.

Several federal emergency management authorities have been invoked for the response to the pandemic, including a presidential declaration of a national emergency, and a declaration by the Secretary of Health and Human Services

* This is an edited, reformatted and augmented edition of a United States Congressional Research Service publication, Report R40554, dated November 16, 2009.

(HHS) of a public health emergency. Among other things, these authorities have allowed federal officials to make certain unapproved drugs available to patients with severe cases of influenza, and to ease certain requirements on hospitals to aid them in caring for surges in the volume of patients.

Federal health officials have purchased millions of doses of H1N1 pandemic flu vaccine, approved through the routine licensing process used for seasonal flu vaccines. A voluntary nationwide vaccination program is underway, largely coordinated by state and local health officials and carried out through public clinics, private health care providers, schools, and others. The Secretary of HHS has implemented waivers of liability and an injury compensation program in the event of unforeseen vaccine safety problems. Allocation schemes were developed to give priority for limited vaccine doses to those in high-risk groups. However, there have been a number of problems associated with shortfalls of actual (versus predicted) vaccine availability, and charges that vaccine would not be available for most of the individuals in designated priority groups until after the peak of pandemic virus transmission had passed. Some Members of Congress and others have questioned the adequacy of federal activities to improve the capacity for and timeliness of flu vaccine production.

To address the outbreak, the Obama Administration requested $2 billion in FY2009 emergency supplemental appropriations, and transfer authority for an additional amount of almost $7 billion from existing HHS accounts. On June 26, the President signed P.L. 111-32, the Supplemental Appropriations Act, 2009, which provided $1.9 billion immediately and an additional $5.8 billion contingent upon a presidential request documenting the need for, and proposed use of, additional funds. The President has subsequently asked for most of the contingent amount. A balance of almost $1.3 billion remains available.

This chapter provides a synopsis of key events in the H1N1 pandemic response, followed by information about selected federal emergency management authorities and actions taken by DHS, HHS, and state and local authorities. It then lists congressional hearings held to date; discusses appropriations and funding for pandemic flu preparedness and response activities; summarizes U.S. government pandemic flu planning documents; and lists sources for additional information. An **Appendix** describes the WHO process to determine the phase of an emerging flu pandemic.

Synopsis

On June 11, 2009, in response to the global spread of a new strain of H1N1 influenza ("flu"), the World Health Organization (WHO) declared the outbreak to be a flu pandemic, the first since 1968. Officials believe the outbreak began in Mexico in March, or perhaps earlier. The novel "H1N1 swine flu" virus was first identified in California in late April. Since then, cases have been reported around the world. The H1N1 pandemic virus is a reassortment of several existing strains of influenza A, subtype H1N1 virus, including strains typically found in pigs, birds, and humans.

Since the H1N1 pandemic virus emerged in the spring, the U.S. Centers for Disease Control and Prevention (CDC) has continued the operation of U.S. seasonal (routine) flu surveillance systems, which are normally suspended during the summer. These systems track trends in rates of illness and hospitalization but are imprecise in their accounting for the total numbers of deaths and hospitalizations due to the pandemic. CDC has published an estimate of these counts, stating that between April and October 17, there were between 14 million and 34 million cases of H1N1 infection, between 63,000 and 153,000 H1N1-related hospitalizations, and between 2,500 and 6,000 H1N1-related deaths in the United States. (See "CDC: Disease Surveillance, and Estimates of Illnesses and Deaths.")

2009 H1N1 Influenza Pandemic Status as of November 16, 2009

International: World Health Organization (WHO):
(http://www.who.int/csr/disease/swineflu/en/index.html)

- WHO declared an influenza pandemic (Phase 6) on June 11. On July 11, WHO asked nations to suspend routine reporting of cases, and stopped publishing case counts, saying they did not accurately reflect pandemic status.
- WHO advises no restriction of regular travel or closure of borders; however, sick individuals are advised to delay travel. Officials report no infection risk from consumption of well-cooked pork products.

United States Government:

(http://www.flu.gov/;http://www.cdc.gov/h1n1flu;http://www.fda.gov/NewsEvents/PublicHealthFocus/ucm150305.htm)

- A Public Health Emergency is in effect under Section 319 of the Public Health Service Act.
- CDC has released to states treatment courses of antiviral drugs, including Tamiflu, Relenza, and the intravenous drug peramivir.
- FDA has issued Emergency Use Authorizations for unapproved uses of Tamiflu and Relenza, use of the unapproved antiviral drug peramivir and unapproved diagnostic tests, and certain uses of protective equipment.
- CDC has issued guidances for the general public; for clinicians and laboratories; regarding pregnant women and other groups; regarding travel; regarding affected schools and communities; and others.
- Congress provided up to $7.7 billion in emergency supplemental appropriations for FY2009 (P.L. 111-32).
- FDA has approved five vaccines against H1N1 flu, through the routine flu vaccine licensing process.
- Health officials have launched a vaccination campaign. HHS Secretary Sebelius has waived liability associated with the use of pandemic vaccine, and enabled an injury compensation program. Priority groups have been identified.
- The President has declared the pandemic to be a national emergency, allowing waivers of some requirements under Medicare and Medicaid law to help health care facilities manage increased numbers of patients.
- CDC estimates that as of October 17, the pandemic had caused between 14 million and 34 million cases of H1N1 infection, between 63,000 and 153,000 H1N1-related hospitalizations, and between 2,500 and 6,000 H1N1-related deaths in the United States.

The CDC reports that the symptoms and transmission of the novel H1N1 flu from person to person are generally similar to seasonal flu. Laboratory testing of the new strain indicates that the antiviral drugs oseltamivir (Tamiflu) and zanamivir (Relenza) are generally effective in treating illnesses caused by the pandemic strain. In contrast to seasonal flu, the pandemic strain appears to cause serious illness more often among children, and less often among the elderly. However, like seasonal flu, pregnant women and individuals with serious chronic diseases appear to be at greater risk of serious illness from the pandemic strain.

In response to the outbreak in April, Janet Napolitano, Secretary of the Department of Homeland Security (DHS), assumed the role of Principal Federal Official, coordinating federal response efforts. Charles E. Johnson, then the Acting Secretary of Health and Human Services (HHS), declared a public health emergency, which remains in effect. Among other things, this has allowed the Food and Drug Administration (FDA) to issue Emergency Use Authorizations (EUAs), permitting certain unapproved uses of antiviral drugs (such as in very young children) and some types of protective facemasks, the use of unapproved diagnostic tests for the new flu strain, and the use of the unapproved antiviral drug peramivir. HHS has established a government-wide informational website (www.flu.gov) with information for planners, health care providers, and the public. On October 24, President Obama declared the pandemic to be a national emergency, which allowed waivers of some requirements under Medicare and Medicaid law to help health care facilities manage increased numbers of patients. To date, there has not been a presidential declaration regarding the pandemic under the Robert T. Stafford Disaster Relief and Emergency Assistance Act (the Stafford Act). The applicability of this Act to infectious disease incidents is unclear. (See "Key Federal Government Authorities and Actions" and **Figure 1**, "Selected Federal Emergency Management Authorities Applicable to the H1N1 Influenza Pandemic.")

Many U.S. communities closed schools when students were found to be infected with the new flu strain. School closure decisions, made by local officials, were based on initial CDC guidance, which was revised as it became clear that the virus was in wide circulation, and that the illnesses it caused were generally mild. CDC now recommends against routine school closures when small numbers of students are infected, arguing that such closures may do little to reduce the spread of the virus, while placing a considerable burden on the affected community. (See "Pandemic Preparedness and Response in Schools.")

The U.S. response to the pandemic triggered a slate of plans that were developed, beginning around 2004, to address concerns about the global spread of another novel flu strain, the H5N1 avian flu. (See box below for definitions.) In FY2006 supplemental appropriations, Congress provided $6.1 billion for pandemic planning across several departments and agencies. These earlier efforts, and others aimed at preparedness for bioterrorism and emerging infections in general, have generally streamlined the response to the H1N1 pandemic. To address the H1N1 outbreak, the Obama Administration requested $2 billion in FY2009 emergency supplemental appropriations, and transfer authority for an additional amount of almost $7 billion from existing HHS accounts. On June 26, the President signed P.L. 111-32, which provided $1.9 billion in FY2009 supplemental appropriations immediately, and an additional $5.8 billion contingent upon a presidential request documenting the need for additional funds. The President has twice requested portions of the contingent funding. (See "Appropriations and Funding.")

INFLUENZA DEFINED

Influenza ("flu") is a respiratory illness that can be transmitted from person to person. Flu viruses are of two main genetic types: Influenza A and B. Influenza A strains are further identified by two important surface proteins that are responsible for virulence: hemagglutinin (H) and neuraminidase (N).

Seasonal flu circulates each year in the winter in each hemisphere. The dominant flu strains in global circulation change from year to year, but most people have some immunity. Infection can be fatal, however. CDC estimates that there are about 36,000 deaths from seasonal flu each year, on average. Vaccines are made each year based on predictions of the strains that are most likely to circulate in the upcoming flu season.

Avian flu ("bird flu") is caused by viruses that occur naturally among wild birds, and that may also affect domestic poultry. In 1997, a new H5N1 strain of avian flu emerged in Asia, and has since caused millions of deaths among domestic poultry, and hundreds of deaths in humans. Health officials have been concerned that this strain could cause a human pandemic, and governments around the world have carried out a number of preparedness activities, including vaccine development and stockpiling, and planning for continuity of services.

Swine flu occurs naturally among wild and domestic swine. People do not normally get swine flu, but each year CDC identifies a few isolated cases of human flu that are caused by flu strains typically associated with swine.

Pandemic flu is caused when a novel strain of human flu (i.e., one that spreads from person to person) emerges and causes a global outbreak, or pandemic, of serious illness. Because there is little natural immunity, the disease is often more severe than is typical of seasonal flu.

(Adapted from HHS, "Flu Terms Defined," *http://www.pandemicflu.gov*. For more information about pandemic flu, see "Understanding Pandemic Influenza" in CRS Report RL33145, *Pandemic Influenza: Domestic Preparedness Efforts*.)

A voluntary national pandemic vaccination campaign is underway. In June, HHS Secretary Kathleen Sebelius issued a declaration waiving liability and enabling a compensation program in the event that injuries result from use of pandemic vaccine. CDC has developed recommendations for groups of individuals who should be given priority for vaccine when it is available in limited amounts. Costs associated with the vaccination program are being funded through both public and private sources. Vaccine is being provided to states as it becomes available, according to states' populations. Vaccine delivery is carried out by a CDC contractor. Decisions regarding vaccine distribution to health care providers, clinics, schools, and other vaccination sites are the responsibility of state and local governments. There have been a number of problems associated with shortfalls of actual (versus predicted) vaccine availability, and charges that vaccine would not be available for most of the individuals in designated priority groups until after the peak of pandemic virus transmission had passed. (See "Vaccines and Pandemic Influenza.")

This chapter provides information about selected federal emergency management authorities and actions taken by DHS and HHS, and actions taken by state and local authorities, in response to the pandemic. It then lists congressional hearings held to date; provides information about appropriations and funding for pandemic flu preparedness and response activities; summarizes U.S. government pandemic flu planning documents; and lists sources for additional information about the pandemic. An **Appendix** describes the WHO process to determine the phase of a threatened or emerging flu pandemic, and touches on several related issues. All dates in this chapter refer to 2009 unless otherwise specified.

KEY FEDERAL GOVERNMENT AUTHORITIES AND ACTIONS

Government-wide Pandemic Preparedness and Response

Leadership and Coordination

Under current law, the Secretary of Homeland Security leads all federal incident response activities, while the Secretary of HHS leads all federal public health and medical incident response activities under the overall leadership of the Secretary of Homeland Security.[1] The Government Accountability Office (GAO) has noted, in the context of pandemic flu planning, that "these federal leadership roles involve shared responsibilities between [HHS] and [DHS], and it is not clear how these would work in practice." GAO recommended that HHS and DHS conduct training and exercises to ensure that federal leadership roles are clearly defined and understood. As recently as July 2009, GAO testified that although some recommended exercises had been undertaken, it was unclear whether they rigorously tested federal leadership roles in a pandemic. GAO also recommended, among other things, that federal pandemic plans published in 2006 be updated.[2] In July, DHS Deputy Secretary Jane Holl Lute testified that an implementation plan for response to the current pandemic was being finalized under the leadership of the National Security Council.[3]

In August, the President's Council of Advisors on Science and Technology (PCAST) released a report assessing preparations for a possible resurgence of H1N1 flu and recommending additional actions.[4] PCAST also noted the potential ambiguity in the leadership roles of DHS and HHS, and recommended that the Homeland Security Advisor[5] be given primary responsibility for decision making during the pandemic response, saying:

> The Working Group has some concerns, based on conversations with representatives of the various agencies involved, that decision-making authorities and processes may not be completely clear in all cases. Primary Federal responsibilities for response to an epidemic are lodged in two departments ([HHS] and DHS), with significant involvement of others (Education, Defense, State, Agriculture, Labor), and coordination by White House staff. While the National Strategy for Pandemic Influenza Implementation Plan provides a comprehensive list of assignments for a multitude of offices, agencies, and departments involved in the Federal planning process, the large number of tasks and responsible units tends to

> obscure the primary seat of responsibility.... The Working Group believes it would be valuable to clarify these matters before events accelerate in September and assign to the Homeland Security Advisor the responsibility for ensuring that all of the important decisions are made in a timely fashion and with appropriate consultation with the President.[6]

Declaration of a National Emergency

On October 23, President Obama declared an emergency, pursuant to the National Emergencies Act, with respect to the H1N1 pandemic. Specifically, the President proclaimed that because "the rapid increase in illness across the nation may overburden health care resources and ... the temporary waiver of certain standard Federal requirements may be warranted in order to enable U.S. health care facilities to implement emergency operations plans, the 2009 H1N1 influenza pandemic in the United States constitutes a national emergency."[7]

The National Emergencies Act provides the President with broad authority to waive statutory requirements, or to invoke other authorities, limited to those he specifies in an emergency declaration. In this case, the declaration was limited to a set of requirements under the Social Security Act, enumerated in Section 1135 of that Act, that may be waived if there are in effect *concurrently* a declaration of public health emergency *and* a presidential declaration under *either* the National Emergencies Act *or* the Robert T. Stafford Disaster Relief and Emergency Assistance Act (the Stafford Act). The National Emergencies Act, the "Section 1135" waiver authority, and other federal emergency management authorities that have been invoked or could be invoked for the response to the flu pandemic are depicted in **Figure 1**. Because a public health emergency declaration was already in effect, the declaration under the National Emergencies Act provided the authority for the Secretary of HHS to waive the Social Security Act requirements in order to make it easier for health care facilities to manage surges in patient volume during the pandemic. The Stafford Act has not been invoked for the response to the H1N1 pandemic. Its possible applicability to this incident is discussed in a subsequent section of this chapter, "Applicability of the Stafford Act." Also, the "Section 1135" waivers are discussed in more detail in a subsequent section, "Waivers or Modifications Under Section 1135 of the Social Security Act."

Department of Homeland Security (DHS)

Leadership Designation

On April 27, Janet Napolitano, Secretary of the Department of Homeland Security (DHS), stated in a press briefing that she was serving as the coordinator of the federal response to the flu outbreak, having assumed the role of Principal Federal Official (PFO).[8] According to the National Response Framework (NRF), which guides a coordinated federal response to disasters and emergencies in general, the Secretary of Homeland Security leads federal incident response.[9]

Applicability of the Stafford Act

As of November 16, the Stafford Act has not been invoked for the response to the H1N1 pandemic. The Act authorizes federal assistance to public and private not-for-profit entities affected by catastrophes, upon a presidential declaration. Two levels of declaration may be made, based on the scope and severity of an incident: a declaration of *emergency*, which provides a lower level of assistance, and a declaration of *major disaster*, which provides a higher level. The Stafford Act is administered by the Federal Emergency Management Agency (FEMA), which can draw from a Disaster Relief Fund to provide assistance for activities that are eligible under the Act.[10]

Major disaster declarations under the Stafford Act have historically involved common meteorological or geological disasters, wildfires, and terrorist acts such as bombings. The applicability of major disaster assistance to infectious disease threats—whether natural (e.g., a flu pandemic) or intentional (bioterrorism)—has been a matter of debate. Historically, major disaster assistance has been tailored to address disaster consequences such as the destruction of infrastructure or the displacement of victims, neither of which is a likely consequence of infectious disease outbreaks.

A legal analysis by CRS concluded that emergency assistance under the Stafford Act could be provided by the President in the event of a flu pandemic, but also noted that whether major disaster assistance would be authorized is not clear. There is no precedent for a major disaster declaration in response to an infectious disease threat. Furthermore, the legislative history of the Stafford Act suggests that this issue was not addressed by Congress when it drafted the current definition of a major disaster, and neither inclusion nor exclusion of flu pandemics from major disaster assistance is required as a matter of statutory construction.[11]

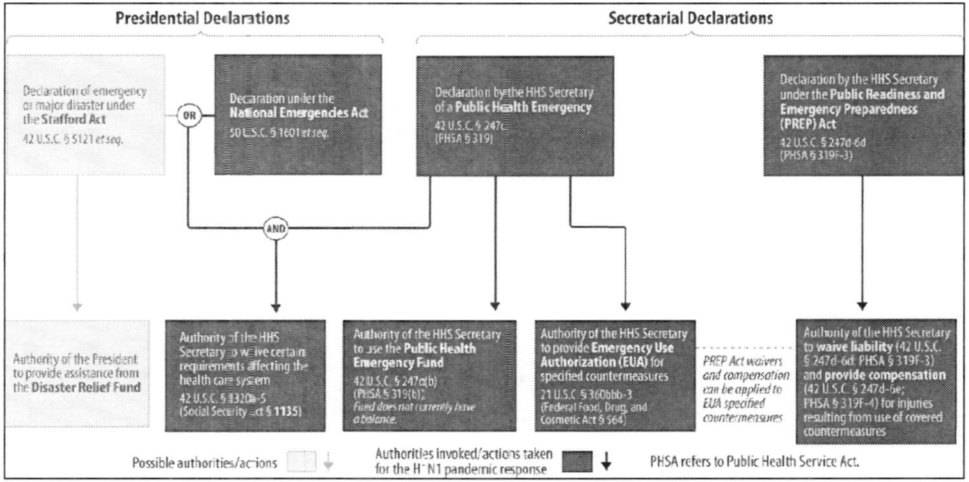

Source: Developed by Congressional Research Service.

Notes: (1) This figure depicts selected authorities that were invoked or could be invoked for the response to the H1N1 flu pandemic, and does not necessarily reflect all available authorities or actions. For example, the National Emergencies Act confers broad authority to the President to waive statutory requirements, or to invoke other authorities, as specified in the declaration of emergency. In this case the declaration was limited to authorities in Section 1135 of the Social Security Act. Similarly, presidential declarations under the Stafford Act may enable authorities, such as certain administrative waivers, in addition to the authority to use the Disaster Relief Fund. (2) The authority for Emergency Use Authorization of specified countermeasures, which was triggered for the H1N1 pandemic by the HHS Secretary's declaration of a public health emergency, can alternatively be triggered by a declaration of a domestic emergency by the Secretary of Homeland Security, or a declaration of a military emergency by the Secretary of Defense. [21 U.S.C. § 360bbb-3(b)]

Figure 1. Selected Federal Emergency Management Authorities Applicable to the H1N1 Influenza Pandemic

In the *National Strategy for Pandemic Influenza: Implementation Plan*, the George W. Bush Administration assumed that the President's authority to declare a major disaster pursuant to the Stafford Act could be applied to a flu pandemic.[12] In 2007, FEMA issued a Disaster Assistance Policy regarding Stafford Act assistance that may be provided during a flu pandemic, which includes costs associated with emergency medical care when provided by an eligible entity (generally, a public or non-profit private entity).[13]

In July, DHS Secretary Janet Napolitano suggested that she did not plan to invoke the Stafford Act for the pandemic response.[14] However, DHS Deputy Secretary Jane Holl Lute has testified that the Stafford Act may be invoked for the pandemic response under certain circumstances, and that DHS has planned accordingly.[15] In information provided by HHS regarding the effects of the presidential declaration of national emergency on October 23, it is suggested that state governors may request that the President make a declaration under the Stafford Act in order to provide assistance if state and local resources become insufficient for the pandemic response.[16] A FEMA fact sheet was referenced in order to assist states in assessing impacts and evaluating the need for federal assistance under the Stafford Act.[17] The Stafford Act and other federal emergency management authorities that have been invoked or could be invoked for the response to the H1N1 flu pandemic are depicted in **Figure 1**.

Customs and Border Protection (CBP) Activities

When the H1N1 flu outbreak began in the United States, Customs and Border Protection (CBP), in DHS, reported monitoring incoming travelers at ports of entry (typically a visual inspection for possible symptoms), providing information about disease control measures, and referring symptomatic persons to a CDC quarantine station[18] or a local public health official for evaluation. According to DHS, "There are no border restrictions in effect. U.S. Customs and Border Protection continues to monitor the health status of incoming visitors at our land, sea and air ports watching out for illness as part of their standard operating procedure."[19]

Administration officials resisted calls for more aggressive measures such as closing the U.S.-Mexico border. WHO and CDC officials commented that scientific evidence does not support closure of a border to travelers as an effective means of controlling the spread of influenza.[20] Also, as a matter of law, U.S. citizens cannot be barred from entering the United States, so any border closure could only exclude aliens.[21] Finally, any such measures would likely be resource-intensive, involving considerable disruption of trade and other economic interests.[22]

Department of Health and Human Services (HHS)

Determination of a Public Health Emergency

On April 26, Charles E. Johnson, then the Acting HHS Secretary, declared a public health emergency pursuant to Section 319 of the Public Health Service Act (PHSA).[23] This enabled FDA to implement an authority in the Federal Food, Drug, and Cosmetic Act (FFDCA) allowing for the emergency use of unapproved medical treatments and tests, under specified conditions, if needed during an incident. (See the subsequent section "FDA: Emergency Use Authorizations.") In addition, while a public health emergency declaration is in effect, the HHS Secretary (or Acting Secretary) is authorized to draw funds for response to the situation from a Public Health Emergency Fund. However, this fund has not had a balance since the 1990s, and hence the declaration did not provide access to this (or any other) emergency funding mechanism. (For more information, see the "Public Health Emergency Funding Mechanisms" section of this chapter.) The public health emergency determination, which would have expired after 90 days, was renewed by HHS Secretary Kathleen Sebelius on July 24 and again on October 1.[24]

The public health emergency authority and other federal emergency management authorities that have been invoked or could be invoked for the response to the H1N1 flu pandemic are depicted in **Figure 1**.

Waivers or Modifications under Section 1135 of the Social Security Act

When there are in effect *concurrently* a declaration of public health emergency *and* a presidential declaration under *either* the National Emergencies Act *or* the Stafford Act, the Secretary of HHS may waive or modify a number of administrative requirements of the Social Security Act and certain health information privacy provisions (as enumerated in Section 1135 of that Act) to streamline the delivery of health care services by facilities facing surges in patient volume.[25] These "1135 waivers" principally involve requirements for reimbursement through the Medicare and Medicaid programs, requirements that most health care facilities in the United States choose to meet.

As noted earlier, on October 23, President Obama declared a national emergency pursuant to the National Emergencies Act. (See the "Declaration of a National Emergency" section of this chapter.) Specifically, the President proclaimed that because "the rapid increase in illness across the nation may overburden health care resources and ... the temporary waiver of certain standard Federal requirements may be warranted in order to enable U.S. health care facilities to implement emergency operations plans, the 2009 H1N1 influenza pandemic in the United States constitutes a national emergency." The President further authorized the Secretary of HHS to "exercise the authority under section 1135 of the Social Security Act to temporarily waive or modify certain requirements of the Medicare, Medicaid, and State Children's Health Insurance programs and of the Health Insurance Portability and Accountability Act [HIPAA] Privacy Rule throughout the duration of the public health emergency declared in response to the 2009 H1N1 influenza pandemic." As noted earlier, a declaration of public health emergency, pursuant to Section 319 of the PHSA, was already in effect.

Section 1135 of the Social Security Act was enacted in the Public Health Security and Bioterrorism Preparedness and Response Act of 2002 (P.L. 107-188). Under this provision, the Secretary may, among other things, waive sanctions under the Emergency Medical Treatment and Active Labor Act (EMTALA) for certain transfers or redirections of patients away from hospital emergency rooms, allowing hospitals to perform triage and direct patients with flu symptoms to alternate facilities set up for that purpose.[26] The Secretary may also waive sanctions and penalties for violations of the HIPAA Privacy Rule in order to facilitate medical recordkeeping when such alternate facilities are used.[27] On October 27, the Secretary of HHS implemented the 1135 waivers, which are administered by the HHS Centers for Medicare and Medicaid Services (CMS).[28]

Waivers under Section 1135 may be applied by the Secretary to any geographic emergency area subject to the concurrent declarations.[29] Waivers have been implemented several times in recent years, beginning with the response to Hurricane Katrina in 2005, pursuant to concurrent public health emergency and Stafford Act declarations. The H1N1 pandemic is the first instance in which the National Emergencies Act, rather than the Stafford Act, was used to enable the 1135 waivers. The "Section 1135" waiver authority and other federal emergency management authorities that have been invoked or could be invoked for the response to the H1N1 flu pandemic are depicted in **Figure 1**.

FDA: Emergency Use Authorizations

If an emerging defense, national security, or public health threat is identified for which no licensed or approved medical product exists, the FFDCA authorizes the FDA Commissioner, under certain conditions, to issue an Emergency Use Authorization (EUA) so that unapproved but potentially helpful countermeasures can be used to protect the public health.[30] Pursuant to authority provided by the public health emergency determination under Section 319 of the PHSA, FDA has issued EUAs to allow emergency use of (1) the antiviral drugs oseltamivir (Tamiflu), zanamivir (Relenza), and peramivir for the treatment or prophylaxis of influenza; (2) disposable respirators for use by the general public; and (3) unapproved diagnostic tests for the new flu strain.[31] Although Tamiflu and Relenza are already approved for use in the United States, the EUAs support federal recommendations to use them in ways not explicitly approved on the product label, such as the use of a product in young children, or beyond a certain duration of a patient's symptoms. Peramivir is an unapproved antiviral drug that can be given intravenously to seriously ill patients (such as patients on ventilators) who are unable to take the oral Tamiflu or inhaled Relenza preparations.

The EUA authority could have been invoked for a pandemic flu vaccine if one had been developed using approaches that are not used in currently licensed products, such as the addition to the vaccine of additives called adjuvants to enhance the immune response. At this time, however, the U.S. government has not purchased H1N1 pandemic vaccines containing adjuvants. All of the government-purchased vaccines have been approved through the routine licensing process used for seasonal flu vaccines. (See the "Pandemic Vaccine Development, Procurement, Production, and Licensing" section of this chapter.) The Emergency Use Authorization and other federal emergency management authorities that have been invoked or could be invoked for the response to the H1N1 flu pandemic are depicted in **Figure 1**.

CDC: Disease Surveillance, and Estimates of Illnesses and Deaths

Because illnesses with the novel H1N1 flu have generally been mild, health officials note that the disease may be substantially underreported. Also, health officials in many U.S. states and cities have stopped running confirmatory tests on suspected cases of H1N1 flu, feeling that better use of epidemiology and laboratory resources can be made by monitoring disease spread to new areas, rather than repeatedly confirming its presence in an affected area.[32]

To get a clearer picture of the spread of H1N1 influenza in the United States, CDC has continued using its multi-layered surveillance system for seasonal flu (which is normally suspended each year in the spring), to which it has added an additional surveillance component to better track the pandemic. (See box below.) On August 30, CDC began accepting reports from states of all influenza- and pneumonia-associated hospitalizations and deaths for the 2009-2010 season. This component tracks both laboratory-confirmed cases of influenza and "syndromic" reports (i.e., cases coded as having pneumonia or influenza whether or not they were laboratory-confirmed as having influenza). Reporting only laboratory-confirmed cases underestimates the burden of illness due to influenza. (Even when testing is done, the test methods have a significant false-negative rate, meaning that the test is negative even though the patient is infected.) In contrast, syndromic reporting captures some cases of pneumonia that are due to causes other than influenza. As CDC notes, although each measure is imperfect, tracking each one nonetheless provides useful information about trends in the spread of the pandemic, and the burdens experienced by the health care system in responding to it.

CDC's Influenza Surveillance Activities

Regular surveillance components used during each annual flu season:

- Viral surveillance, which monitors the percentage of specimens tested for flu that are positive; the types and subtypes of flu viruses circulating; resistance to antiviral medications; and the emergence of new flu strains.
- Selected physician surveillance for influenza-like illness (ILI), which monitors the percentage of visits for symptoms that could be the flu.
- Hospitalization surveillance, which tracks numbers of hospitalizations with laboratory-confirmed flu infections among adults and children.
- Summary of the geographic spread of flu, which tracks the number of states affected by flu, and the degree to which they are affected.
- Deaths from 122 cities that report the total number of deaths and the percentage of those that are coded as influenza or pneumonia.
- The number of laboratory-confirmed deaths from flu among children.

Added surveillance component for the H1N1 flu pandemic:

- Reports by states of either laboratory-confirmed hospitalizations and deaths from flu, or syndromic cases, i.e. cases of presumed influenza and/or pneumonia based on ICD-9 coded hospitalizations or death reports.

Source: Adapted from CDC, "Reporting of Influenza and Pneumonia-Associated Hospitalizations and Deaths for the 2009-2010 Season," September 11, 2009, http://www.cdc.gov/h1n1flu/reportingqa.htm#surveillancesystems.

According to CDC, "Routine seasonal surveillance does not count individual flu cases, hospitalizations or deaths (except for pediatric influenza deaths) but instead monitors activity levels and trends and virus characteristics through a nationwide surveillance system."[33] Except for pediatric deaths, the surveillance mechanisms currently available do not provide health officials with an accurate count of deaths attributable to the pandemic. Instead, officials derive estimates from a number of available sources of information, and these estimates are generally considered to reflect mortality more accurately than do "case counts." On November 12, CDC published a comprehensive estimate of the burden of illness caused by the H1N1 pandemic in the United States, stating that between April, when the novel flu strain was first identified, and October 17, there were between 14 million and 34 million cases of H1N1 infection; between 63,000 and 153,000 H1N1-related hospitalizations; and between 2,500 and 6,000 H1N1-related deaths in the United States.[34] CDC says it plans to update these estimates every three to four weeks.

CDC's surveillance systems showed that during the week ending November 7, 2009, all of the typed flu viruses reported nationwide were the H1N1 pandemic strain. Thirty-five influenza-associated pediatric deaths were reported, the highest weekly total since the pandemic began. Almost all of the flu viruses tested were sensitive to the antiviral drug Tamiflu. Forty-six states reported widespread influenza activity. Indicators in some regions of the country showed evidence of increasing transmission of the virus, while indicators in some other regions showed declines from previous weeks.[35]

VACCINES AND PANDEMIC INFLUENZA

The 2009 H1N1 Pandemic Vaccine Program

In September, the FDA licensed four vaccines against the H1N1 pandemic flu strain. (A fifth vaccine was licensed in November.) As vaccine became available in early October, federal, state, and local health officials began a voluntary nationwide vaccination campaign, which some have said is the most extensive such effort ever undertaken in the United States. This section discusses the production of the H1N1 pandemic vaccines, various activities involved in conducting the pandemic vaccination program, and associated issues.

Overview

Vaccination is considered the best preventive measure against influenza. But, because of continuous changes in the genes of flu viruses, vaccines must be "matched" to strains in circulation to provoke good immunity, and new vaccines must be developed for each year's flu season.

In the United States, all currently licensed seasonal flu vaccines are produced using a time-consuming process involving specially raised, fertilized hen's eggs. First, the virus is adapted for mass production and suitability for use in a vaccine. (The adapted virus is called a "seed" virus.) Next, the seed virus is grown in the eggs in large amounts. Next, small amounts of finished vaccine are produced for use in clinical trials. Finally, if trials demonstrate that the vaccine is safe and effective, then finished vaccine is mass produced.[36] Production capacity is finite, so vaccine becomes available in batches. To develop vaccine for a typical Northern Hemisphere flu season, three flu strains are selected in January or February of each year (based on strains circulating in the Southern Hemisphere). Vaccine is produced and becomes available over the next six to nine months, typically from September through December of each year, before the peak of each flu season. Adapting and growing the virus can take variable amounts of time, and different flu strains "behave" differently during this process. In the best case, all of the steps described above take at least four months. More typically, at least six months is required.

Because flu vaccines cannot be produced until the strains they would protect against are in circulation, it was essential, when the H1N1 pandemic was first recognized in late April, to begin development of a vaccine immediately. Although the new flu strain caused illnesses and deaths across the United States from the time it first emerged, it would be months before any vaccine made using current production methods would be available to protect against it.

Recent U.S. pandemic planning efforts have focused on (1) expanding domestic capacity to mass-produce flu vaccine in the near term; (2) developing approaches to speed up and "stretch" existing production capacity, such as through the use of *adjuvants,* vaccine additives that boost the immune response so that a lower virus dose is effective;[37] and (3) developing better approaches for flu vaccine production in the future. Although recent progress has been made to improve domestic production capacity, the vaccines developed for use in the United States against the H1N1 pandemic strain use the egg-based process, with its significant lag time.

Pandemic Vaccine Development, Procurement, Production, and Licensing

This section discusses influenza vaccine development, procurement, production, and licensing for the H1N1 pandemic. Issues related to improving future influenza vaccine production capacity are discussed in a later section of this chapter, "Ways to Improve Influenza Vaccine Production in the Future."

Federal officials have said that there are three key decision points in developing and using pandemic flu vaccines: (1) to develop adapted "seed" viruses and a prototype vaccine(s), and to conduct clinical trials; (2) to purchase and mass-produce large amounts of a promising vaccine; and (3) to administer the vaccine widely, that is, to conduct a mass-vaccination campaign. These decision points are presented in a timeline of the U.S. pandemic flu vaccine strategy in **Figure 2**. The figure also shows that a second wave of heightened transmission of H1N1 flu in the United States in the fall could precede the peak of seasonal flu activity and the initial availability of pandemic vaccine. Finally, the figure shows the overlap between the production of seasonal flu vaccine for the Northern Hemisphere and production of H1N1 pandemic vaccine.

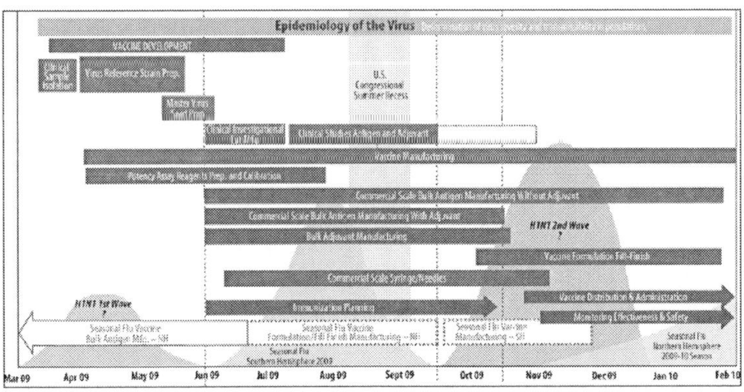

Source: Adapted by CRS from background material provided for a meeting of the National Biodefense Science Board (administered by HHS) regarding the U.S. 2009 H1N1 vaccine strategy, May 22, 2009, *http://www.hhs.gov/aspr/conferences/nbsb/090522-nbsb-meeting.html*.

Figure 2. Timeline for H1N1 Pandemic Vaccine Development, Manufacturing, and Possible Distribution and Administration

Over the spring and summer, HHS issued purchase orders for H1N1 pandemic vaccine, based on existing contracts with producers of seasonal flu vaccines that are currently licensed in the United States.[38] Development and procurement efforts are led by the HHS Biomedical Advanced Research and Development Authority (BARDA), in coordination with the National Institutes of Health (NIH), FDA, CDC, and other HHS agencies.

The NIH National Institute of Allergy and Infectious Diseases (NIAID) is responsible for coordinating clinical trials to determine safety, effectiveness, and optimum dosing for the H1N1 pandemic vaccine.[39] Trials conducted in late summer on healthy adults yielded favorable results. First, the same dose of virus that is used in seasonal flu vaccines was protective when used for the pandemic vaccine. Second, one pandemic vaccine provided protection in adults; a "booster" would not be needed. Third, no serious safety concerns were noted. As a result, large numbers of pandemic vaccines could be produced with existing capacity. Also, adjuvants would not be used, which meant that pandemic vaccines could be evaluated for licensing through the usual process for seasonal flu vaccines; namely, as amendments to the existing product licenses. Emergency Use Authorizations would not be necessary. (See the prior section, "FDA: Emergency Use Authorizations," for more information about this authority.) H1N1 vaccine clinical trials on children, pregnant women, and individuals with HIV are also underway or have been completed. Finally, NIAID has begun clinical trials on H1N1 vaccines containing adjuvant. Officials have said that although they do not think that adjuvanted vaccine will be needed for the domestic pandemic vaccination program, it could be useful to have the option to use adjuvanted vaccine if the virus mutates to a different form (potentially rendering the non-adjuvanted vaccines less effective). They have also said that research on adjuvants contributes to the knowledge base to improve influenza vaccine production in general.

On September 16, FDA announced that it had approved H1N1 pandemic flu vaccines made by four companies: Sanofi Pasteur Inc., CSL Limited, Novartis Vaccines and Diagnostics Limited, and MedImmune LLC.[40] On November 10, FDA approved a fifth pandemic vaccine made by ID Biomedical Corporation of Quebec, a subsidiary of GlaxoSmithKline. The Medimmune product is an intranasal vaccine. The other four products are injectable vaccines. The approved uses of each product vary somewhat. In general, for the injectable vaccines, healthy adults should receive one dose, and children aged six months to nine years of age should receive two, in order to raise protective immunity. None of the products is approved for use in infants under six months of age. The approved uses for the intranasal vaccine are more narrow than for the injectable products. In general, the intranasal vaccine is approved for use in healthy individuals aged 2 to 49 years. None of the products contains an adjuvant. The injectable products are available in both multi-dose vials containing a preservative, and in single-dose syringes without a preservative.[41]

Vaccine Financing[42]

Congress provided up to $7.65 billion in FY2009 supplemental appropriations to HHS for the pandemic response, part of which has been used to support the purchase of vaccine and associated costs of planning and carrying out a nationwide vaccination campaign. (See the subsequent section "Emergency Supplemental Appropriations for FY2009.") There are two types of costs associated with furnishing vaccinations to individuals: the costs of the vaccine and associated supplies, and the costs for administration of the vaccine, which typically include the value of a provider's time, costs for refrigerated storage and recordkeeping, and related costs.

According to CDC, all pandemic flu vaccines and necessary supplies—syringes, needles, sharps containers, and alcohol swabs—have been purchased by the federal government and are being made available to vaccinators across the country at no cost. In no case may a provider or insurer charge individuals for these costs. Plans for payment of administration costs vary. Medicare, the Department of Veterans Affairs, and many private insurers have said they will cover the costs of administration for seasonal flu vaccine and one or more pandemic vaccines. Private providers (including physicians and chain pharmacies) may charge appropriate fees for the costs of administration if public or private insurance is not available, or they may waive these fees. States are expected to use a portion of the federal funds they received for pandemic planning to support clinics at which individuals who are uninsured can be vaccinated without charge. Also, Federally Qualified Health Centers are expected to provide services, including vaccination for pandemic flu, regardless of ability to pay.

Vaccine Distribution[43]

Federal officials are working with state and local health officials to implement a "blended" public- and private-sector distribution approach to provide pandemic vaccines to any individuals who want to be vaccinated. During each flu season, much of the vaccine is purchased and delivered through private-sector distributors and providers. For the response to unanticipated threats such as bioterrorism, CDC maintains the Strategic National Stockpile (SNS) of drugs and medical supplies, and provides training and technical assistance to state and local health officials, who are responsible for distribution of stockpile materiel within their jurisdictions. Under the Vaccines for Children program, CDC distributes recommended pediatric vaccines (financed by the Medicaid program) to private providers for administration to eligible low-income children. The blended approach being used for the pandemic vaccination campaign uses portions of each of these mechanisms to make vaccine available to a variety of public- and private-sector providers and clinics. To distribute vaccine as it becomes available, CDC has contracted with McKesson Corporation, the agency's contractor for distribution under the Vaccines for Children program.[44]

In early October, limited amounts of the approved intranasal H1N1 pandemic vaccine became available and were provided to states according to their populations. Available amounts were less than expected, posing problems for many states and localities, which had planned to conduct or coordinate vaccination clinics based on projected vaccine availability.[45] In August, CDC reported expecting "... somewhere between 45 million and 52 million doses of vaccine to be available by mid-October. This will be followed by weekly availability of vaccine up to about 195 million doses by the end of the year."[46] In mid-October, CDC reported that only 11.4 million doses of the injectable H1N1 vaccine were available.[47] CDC said that manufacturers were experiencing several problems that affected production volume, including slower than expected growth of the virus in eggs.

Despite high demand for the vaccine, some states appear to have had difficulty getting available vaccine into distribution in their jurisdictions. The distribution plan calls on states to "order" vaccine from their allotments when they are ready to direct how it is to be distributed within the state. HHS publishes daily updates of the total (national) amounts of vaccine *allocated* (i.e., available to states), *ordered* by states, and actually *shipped*, as well as daily updates of the number of vaccines shipped to each state.[48] Because vaccine is allocated to states according to population, calculating the number of vaccines shipped to each state according to its population should yield similar ratios if the states are similar in their efficiency at ordering and directing the distribution of vaccine within their jurisdictions. However, a news organization has published such an analysis and found considerable variation among the states.[49]

Despite some statements to the contrary, the civilian vaccination program for the H1N1 pandemic is voluntary. There have been no plans at the federal, state, or local level to require that members of the general public be vaccinated. However, requirements have been established by the Department of Defense, and by some states and private health systems, for the vaccination of health care workers. Public health officials recommend that health care workers be vaccinated against influenza (including pandemic flu) not only for their own protection, but also in order to protect patients from infection by their providers, and to prevent levels of absenteeism among providers that could threaten the quality of patient care.[50]

Allocation to Priority Groups[51]

CDC advises that anyone who wishes to be vaccinated for seasonal and/or pandemic influenza should seek the vaccine(s) when adequate supplies are available. Certain groups are especially advised to be vaccinated due to their risk of more serious complications from influenza, the risk that they would transmit influenza to others, or both. These groups, identified by the Advisory Committee on Immunization Practices (ACIP, which advises the CDC Director), are

- pregnant women;
- persons who live with or provide care for infants aged less than 6 months (e.g., parents, siblings, and daycare providers), because these infants cannot receive the vaccine;
- health-care and emergency medical services personnel;
- persons aged 6 months-24 years; and
- persons aged 25-64 years who have medical conditions that put them at higher risk for influenza-related complications.[52]

ACIP estimated that the five groups above comprise about 159 million persons in the United States.

Because the H1N1 pandemic vaccine is becoming available in phases, initial demand has exceeded supply. Anticipating this, ACIP also identified a subset of these groups that should be given priority when vaccine supplies are limited. These priority groups are

- pregnant women (as above);
- persons who live with or provide care for infants aged less than 6 months (as above);

- health-care and emergency medical services personnel who have direct contact with patients or infectious material (a subset of the recommended group above);
- children aged 6 months-4 years (only the youngest children); and
- children and adolescents aged 5-18 years who have medical conditions that put them at higher risk for influenza-related complications (only children with medical conditions, versus all persons under age 65 with medical conditions).[53]

ACIP estimated that this subset of priority groups comprises about 42 million persons in the United States.

Available vaccine may be either the injectable or intranasal formulation. In general, injectable H1N1 vaccine may be given to anyone in one of the priority groups who does not have a specific contraindication (such as an allergy to eggs). However, the intranasal vaccine is not licensed for use in some individuals within the pandemic priority groups. Prioritized individuals who should not receive the intranasal vaccine include pregnant women, children younger than two years of age, individuals of any age who have chronic illnesses, and health care workers who care for severely immunocompromised patients, such as those who have recently undergone bone marrow transplantation. Although federal authorities provide guidance on vaccine allocation, final allocation decisions, and any enforcement of them, is made at the state and local levels.[54]

Adverse Event Monitoring[55]

Although clinical trials were conducted on the approved H1N1 pandemic vaccines and did not show any serious adverse events (i.e., side effects), rare adverse events would not necessarily manifest until a product was widely used. Health officials plan to monitor for any possible adverse events among persons who receive the H1N1 pandemic vaccine, using, among other approaches, the existing Vaccine Adverse Event Reporting System (VAERS), a national vaccine safety surveillance program co-sponsored by CDC and FDA. VAERS accepts reports from patients, providers, public health officials, and others through a website and toll-free number.[56]

In 1976, a U.S. vaccination campaign was carried out for a pandemic flu threat that did not materialize (also called "Swine Flu"). However, evidence suggested that among those vaccinated, there may have been an increased risk of a serious and sometimes fatal neurologic side effect, a form of paralysis called Guillain-Barre Syndrome (GBS). The vaccination campaign was called off, and the credibility of public health officials was significantly compromised by the incident.[57]

Liability and Compensation

On June 25, HHS Secretary Kathleen Sebelius issued a declaration under the Public Readiness and Emergency Preparedness Act (PREP Act, Division C of P.L. 109-148) regarding the H1N1 pandemic vaccine.[58] The PREP Act waives liability and establishes an injury compensation program for the use of certain "covered countermeasures." The June 25 declaration eliminates liability (with the exception of willful misconduct) for the United States, and for manufacturers, distributors, program planners, persons who prescribe, and employees of any of the above, who administer or dispense an H1N1 pandemic vaccine that qualifies as a "covered countermeasure" under conditions specified by the Secretary in the declaration.[59] Under the law, claims under state law are preempted. As noted in **Figure 1**, authorities under the PREP Act are independent from other emergency authorities that have been invoked for the response to the H1N1 pandemic.[60]

In addition to the limitation of liability, the PREP Act declaration also establishes a federal program to compensate individuals who are vaccinated for any serious injuries or death that occurs as a result of the H1N1 vaccine, and authority for a fund to pay claims. The compensation program is administered by the HHS Health Resources and Services Administration (HRSA), using the Smallpox Vaccine Injury Compensation Program as an administrative model.[61] The fund, called the Covered Countermeasure Process Fund (CCPF), did not have a balance of funds when the H1N1 pandemic began. However, in providing emergency supplemental funding for pandemic preparedness (P.L. 111-32), Congress authorized the use of an unspecified amount of the appropriation for the CCPF.[62] On July 16, President Obama requested additional contingent funding under the new law, to be used for several activities, including funding for the CCPF.[63]

Ways to Improve Influenza Vaccine Production in the Future

Strengths and Limitations of Egg-Based Technology

In its 2005 strategy for influenza pandemic preparedness, the George W. Bush Administration set a goal to "establish domestic production capacity to ensure ... [s]ufficient vaccine to vaccinate the entire U.S. population within six months of the emergence of a virus with pandemic potential."[64] Because a flu pandemic could emerge at any time, federal officials saw this as a multi-pronged strategy, requiring concurrent investments in the expansion of production capacity using current approaches, and in the development of new approaches.

In January 2009, when announcing federal funding for a new private facility to manufacture cell-based influenza vaccine, an HHS official said that the strategic goal above " ... could not be accomplished using the traditional egg-based method of producing flu vaccine."[65] Nonetheless, significant federal investments were made to expand production capacity for egg-based vaccine in the event that a flu pandemic arose in the near term. Although concerns were largely driven at the time by the spread of H5N1 avian flu, it was the surprising emergence of H1N1 pandemic flu that proved to be the test of the federal strategy.

Investments to date have had mixed results. The United States has ordered H1N1 pandemic vaccine sufficient to provide 250 million doses, representing substantially greater total capacity than was available only several years ago. Yet the lag time inherent in egg-based vaccine technology is unavoidable, and its effects are stark as the H1N1 pandemic unfolds in a largely unimmunized population. Several observers have suggested that peak nationwide transmission of the virus will have occurred before substantial amounts of vaccine are available.[66]

Some have suggested that even though the lag time to first vaccine availability was unavoidable, there could have been more investment or better planning for the use of egg-based vaccine to avoid the shortage that persists more than a month into the vaccination campaign. For example, some assert that the decision to forgo the use of adjuvants in the pandemic vaccine was made when officials were more optimistic about a timely roll-out of the product, and that more vaccine doses would now be available if adjuvant had been used. However, there are no adjuvant-containing seasonal flu vaccines currently licensed in the United States, so the use of this approach for the pandemic would have required Emergency Use Authorization of the vaccine, which could well have delayed its availability. The use of adjuvants and an emergency licensing process could also have contributed to apprehensions among the public about the vaccine's safety.

Strengths and Limitations of Cell-Based Technology

Other observers assert that greater investment in cell-based (rather than egg-based) vaccine technology could potentially have made that approach viable for the response to the H1N1 pandemic, and that the current vaccination program could have been farther along in that case. In the cell-based approach, the influenza virus is grown in one of a number of types of cells, which are generally easier to manage on the industrial scale than is growth in eggs. The European Medicines Agency (EMEA) licensed a cell-based seasonal influenza vaccine, Optaflu, in 2007, and has also licensed a cell-based H1N1 pandemic vaccine, Celvapan.[67]

However, an HHS official, among others, has noted that cell-based approaches to the production of influenza vaccine are not likely to substantially shorten the time to first vaccine availability, compared with egg-based production, because the process still requires growing whole influenza virus in the cells.[68] Rather, the advantage of cell-based over egg-based production in the near term is one of scalability, or "throughput" (i.e., once virus is grown, vaccines can be finished in large quantities quickly, making hundreds of millions of doses available within weeks rather than months from the time the first batches become available). With egg-based approaches, the dependence on specially produced fertilized eggs limits this scalability. If cell-based approaches had been available for the response to the H1N1 pandemic, it is possible that more vaccine could have been finished by this point, although it still might not have first become available until several months into the pandemic, as was the case with the egg-based vaccines in use.

Recombinant, DNA-Based, and Other Advanced Technologies

Alternative approaches under development for the production of flu vaccine involve technologies that do not require the use of whole viruses (therefore eliminating the need to grow them), but rather focus on producing only those portions (subunits) of the virus that are needed to produce immunity, such as a particular protein in the virus coat. For example, using *recombinant* technology, the genes for the desired virus subunit may be inserted into another microorganism that grows well, such as yeast. The subunit is then replicated by the host microorganism, harvested, purified, and made into a vaccine containing only the subunit, not whole virus. Another recombinant approach places the genes for the desired virus subunit into another virus (called a vector) that introduces the subunit into the body, but does not itself cause disease. More sophisticated approaches to vaccine production involve making *DNA-based* vaccines consisting solely of the viral genes.[69] The "Holy Grail" for the prevention of influenza is the so-called *universal* influenza vaccine, one that could be administered in childhood to protect against whatever variations of seasonal or pandemic flu arise throughout one's lifetime.

Federal Efforts to Improve Influenza Vaccine Technology

All U.S.-licensed seasonal and pandemic flu vaccines are made using the whole virus, egg-based approach. As noted earlier, cell-based whole virus influenza vaccines have been licensed in Europe. Recombinant vaccines that have been licensed for use in the United States include those against hepatitis B and human papillomavirus. There has not yet been a DNA-based vaccine licensed for use in humans in the United States or Europe. Each of these approaches to vaccine production, including the production of influenza vaccine, is also applied in licensed or investigational products for veterinary uses in animals.

The NIH provides federal leadership for basic biomedical research on promising vaccine technologies. A search of the NIH ClinicalTrials.gov database yielded a number of clinical trials—in progress or completed—on influenza vaccine prototypes developed using recombinant techniques. The trials range from Phase I—the earliest stage of investigation involving small numbers of human subjects—to Phase III trials involving large numbers of subjects.[70] In addition, several Phase I trials of DNA-based influenza vaccines were found. In FY2008, NIH reported spending $204 million on influenza research, including a number of projects specifically involving advanced approaches to influenza vaccine production, and research on other aspects of influenza immunology that are applicable to vaccine development.[71] NIH has also sponsored many clinical trials of vaccines against H1N1 pandemic flu, as well as H5N1 avian and other flu strains, for the purposes of licensing and/or stockpiling these vaccines.[72] Federal leadership for advanced development of emergency medical countermeasures, including pandemic products, is provided by the Biomedical Advanced Research and Development Authority (BARDA), in HHS. Federal investments in the advanced development of flu vaccine technology came principally from FY2006 emergency supplemental funds for pandemic preparedness,[73] and were administered by BARDA. (See the subsequent section "Prior Funding for Pandemic Flu Preparedness.") HHS has published several reports, as required by Congress, detailing the use of these funds. **Table 1** presents funding amounts for pandemic vaccine development activities, as reported by HHS in January 2009. The focus of this spending has been on expanding egg-based and cell-based vaccine production capacity, as these approaches were clearly viable to make products that could be licensed for use in the United States.

Table 1. FY2006 Supplemental Funding for Pandemic Influenza Vaccine Activities Obligations, Dollars in Millions, as of December 31, 2008

Activity	Amount
Egg-based vaccine capacity and purchases[a]	875.7
Retrofit existing facilities for emergency production[b]	121.0
Accelerate cell-based vaccine[c]	1,707.3
Advanced development of antigen-sparing techniques[d]	155.6
FDA activities[e]	20
SUBTOTAL, obligations for vaccine activities	2879.5
Unobligated funds for vaccine activities	316.5
TOTAL, allocations for vaccine activities	**3,196.0**

Source: Prepared by Congressional Research Service from HHS, Assistant Secretary for Resources and Technology, "Report to Congress: Pandemic Influenza Preparedness Spending," Table, pp. 16-17, January 2009, *http://www.hhs.gov/aspr/barda/mcm/panflu/spending.html*.

Notes: Numbers do not add due to rounding.

a. Includes funds for contracts with Chiron, GlaxoSmithKline, Novartis, and Sanofi Pasteur for purchase and maintenance of vaccine against H5N1 avian flu.

b. Includes funds for contracts with Medimmune and Sanofi Pasteur.

c. Includes funds for contracts with Dynport, GlaxoSmithKline, Medimmune, Novartis, and Solvay.

d. Includes funds for several contracts to study use of adjuvants.

e. Includes funds to expand regulatory capacity, including laboratory expansion and supplies, information technology support, program management, and other activities.

Along with contracts to purchase vaccine from companies developing these products, HHS funds have also been used to construct or retrofit domestic vaccine production facilities. As noted earlier, the national strategic goal for pandemic preparedness was the establishment of sufficient *domestic* flu vaccine production capacity. To this end, HHS funds were provided to Sanofi Pasteur and Medimmune to expand their domestic facilities for egg-based vaccine production.[74]

In addition, HHS has awarded a $487 million contract to Novartis Vaccines and Diagnostics, Inc., to build a facility in North Carolina to make cell-based seasonal and pandemic flu vaccine.[75]

In April 2009, before the emergence of the H1N1 pandemic flu strain, BARDA announced an upcoming Request for Proposals (RFP) for advanced development of recombinant influenza vaccine products for both seasonal and pandemic use, which would provide federal funding to advance the commercial development of this technology. In its presolicitation notice, HHS said

> The timeline for the availability of egg- and cell-based inactivated [i.e., whole virus] pandemic influenza vaccines in the U.S. is estimated at 20-23 weeks post-pandemic onset, which may be towards the end of a first pandemic wave. Recombinant influenza vaccines, on the other hand, may benefit from manufacturing efficiencies, may not be dependent on pandemic influenza virus reference strain availability and/or the production and calibration of potency assay reagents needed for inactivated influenza vaccines. As a result, recombinant influenza vaccines may be available in a shorter time frame of 8 to 12 weeks post-pandemic onset. The effect of vaccination combined with influenza antiviral drugs and community mitigation measures may delay the peak incidence of pandemic influenza disease and reduce mortality and morbidity during a severe pandemic.[76]

In response to questions about the RFP above, HHS commented that it intends that successful applicants would pursue approaches applicable to both seasonal and pandemic flu vaccine production. There are obvious advantages to using a tried-and-true approach in an emergency (i.e., basing pandemic flu vaccine production on the approach used to make seasonal flu vaccine). Egg-based seasonal flu vaccine is a safe, inexpensive, and widely accepted product. A possible disadvantage of changing to a different approach is that seasonal flu vaccine could become more costly, at least initially. An HHS official, when asked whether use of cell-based and newer production methods could make seasonal flu vaccine more costly, replied that new technologies were likely to be more expensive initially.[77] Although there has been little public debate about this, an increase in the cost of seasonal flu vaccine could have consequences for public health efforts to expand the utilization of this product.

Key State and Local Pandemic Response Activities

State Pandemic Preparedness and Response

Since FY2002, all states have received HHS funds to prepare their public health and health care systems for public health threats and emergencies.[78]

Beginning with FY2004, states were required, as a condition of these funds, to develop plans specifically for the response to a flu pandemic. Subsequently, Congress provided $600 million in FY2006 emergency supplemental appropriations for states to continue their pandemic planning efforts.[79] When the H1N1 flu outbreak emerged, Congress provided an additional $350 million in FY2009 emergency supplemental appropriations for state pandemic response.[80] (See the subsequent section "Emergency Supplemental Appropriations for FY2009.")

Based on an analysis of state pandemic flu plans available as of July 2006, CRS found the plans to be more robust in their discussion of core public health activities such as disease surveillance and laboratory activities, and less robust in aspects of multi-sector preparedness, such as leadership designation, incident management, certain aspects of health care surge planning, and continuity planning for essential services such as food distribution.[81]

In January 2009, HHS and DHS published *Assessment of States' Operating Plans to Combat Pandemic Influenza: Report to Homeland Security Council* (state assessment report), the findings of their comprehensive joint assessment of state pandemic planning through 2008.[82] This assessment echoed the findings of CRS, saying that preparedness was most advanced with respect to objectives that are exclusively or primarily the responsibility of state public health agencies, namely infectious disease surveillance and clinical laboratory operations; distribution of antiviral drugs and vaccines; mass vaccination; and public communications. In contrast, the assessment found that states were having difficulty planning for surges in health care and emergency medical services, and were especially having difficulty planning for continuity of non-health services, such as continuity of state agency operations; coordination of military support to civil authorities; law enforcement continuity; and ensuring the safety of the food supply.

Thus far, dedicated federal funding to state and local governments for pandemic preparedness has been provided only through HHS grants. Noting the challenges states face in assuring preparedness in non-health sectors, the state assessment report comments, "The [U.S. Government] has provided guidance and technical assistance for many of these activities but generally has not been in a position to award funds to help States develop them in the context of pandemic influenza preparedness."[83]

If the pandemic continues to unfold as it has, producing generally mild to moderate illness, the pandemic's effects on non-health sectors such as transportation and public utilities could be minimal. However, despite the high marks for mass vaccination planning received by most states in the state assessment report, considerable public attention has focused on apparent delays by some states in ordering available vaccine from CDC and promptly distributing it.[84]

Pandemic Preparedness and Response in Schools[85]

When the H1N1 outbreak first began in the United States, some affected communities closed schools when students were found to be infected. Legal authority to close schools rests with state or local officials and is highly variable among the states. A CDC-requested study found that school closure is legally possible in most jurisdictions during both routine and emergency situations.[86] The study also indicated that state authority for closure may be vested at various levels of government and in different departments, generally the state or local education agencies or state or local departments of health.

When the H1N1 pandemic first emerged in the spring, CDC, in consultation with the U.S. Department of Education, issued guidance with respect to school closures (based on earlier guidance from 2007), recommending that "affected communities with laboratory-confirmed cases of influenza A H1N1 consider adopting school dismissal and childcare closure measures, including closing for up to 14 days depending on the extent and severity of illness."[87] School closures are challenging for all parties involved. Among other things, parents must find alternate arrangements for care of their children, educators must adopt alternate means of delivering their services, and children's education may be compromised. On May 5, CDC officials reissued their guidance regarding school closures, recommending against closures based on individual cases of H1N1 flu. It recommended instead that emphasis be placed on keeping sick students and employees home, and that closings be considered if absenteeism was substantial.[88]

As with CDC guidance in general, recommendations regarding school closure are intended to be weighed by local officials in light of local circumstances. In addition to uncertainty about the outbreak's initial severity, there may also have been uncertainty among state and local officials about decision-making protocols. In an assessment of state pandemic flu preparedness conducted by HHS and DHS in 2007 through 2008, planning for student dismissal and school closure was found to be a weakness among the states. More than half of them were graded as having either "many major gaps" or "inadequate preparedness" for this planning task.[89]

Outbreaks in schools largely subsided over the summer. Transmission of the H1N1 virus reemerged in a number of elementary and secondary schools and in colleges and universities as students returned for the fall. The American College Health Association (ACHA) began tracking voluntary reports of pandemic flu activity at colleges and universities.[90] For the week ending November 6, ACHA saw sustained high levels of nationwide reporting of influenza-like illnesses. Reporting was on the decline in many states, however.

CONGRESSIONAL HEARINGS

Congressional committees in both chambers have convened hearings to assess the emergence of the new strain of H1N1 influenza. Hearings are listed in **Table 2**.

Table 2. Congressional Hearings on the 2009 Influenza Pandemic

Date	Committee (/Subcommittee)	Topic
SENATE		
Apr. 28, 2009	Appropriations / Labor, HHS, Education, and Related Agencies	The Public Health Response to the Swine Flu Epidemic
Apr. 29, 2009	Health, Education, Labor, and Pensions (HELP)	The Swine Flu Epidemic: The Public Health and Medical Response
Apr. 29, 2009	Homeland Security and Governmental Affairs Committee (HSGAC)	Swine Flu: Coordinating the Federal Response
May 7, 2009	Appropriations / Agriculture, Rural Development, and FDA	Hearing to Discuss the 2009 H1N1 Virus
June 3, 2009	HSGAC / State, Local and Private Sector Preparedness and Integration	Pandemic Flu: Closing the Gaps
June 16, 2009	HSGAC / Oversight of Government Management, the Federal Workforce and District of Columbia	Pandemic Flu Preparedness and the Federal Workforce
Sept. 21, 2009	HSGAC	H1N1 Flu: Protecting Our Community[a]

Table 2. (Continued)

Date	Committee (/Subcommittee)	Topic
Oct. 21, 2009	HSGAC	H1N1 Flu: Monitoring the Nation's Response
Nov. 10, 2009	HELP / Children and Families	The Cost of Being Sick: H1N1 and Paid Sick Days
Nov. 17, 2009	HSGAC	H1N1 Flu: Getting the Vaccine to Where It Is Needed Most
HOUSE		
Apr. 30, 2009	Energy and Commerce / Health	Swine Flu Outbreak and the U.S. Federal Response
May 6, 2009	Foreign Affairs / Africa and Global Health	Global Health Emergencies Hit Home: The Swine Flu Outbreak
May 7, 2009	Education and Labor	Ensuring Preparedness Against the Flu Virus at School and Work
May 14, 2009	Oversight and Government Reform/Federal Workforce, Postal Service, and the District of Columbia	Protecting the Protectors: An Assessment of Front-Line Federal Workers in Response to the H1N1 Flu
May 20, 2009	Oversight and Government Reform	State and Local Pandemic Preparedness
July 29, 2009	Homeland Security	Beyond Readiness: An Examination of the Current Status and Future Outlook of the National Response to Pandemic Influenza
Sept. 9, 2009	Small Business	The Challenges of the 2009-H1N1 Influenza and its Potential Impact on Small Businesses and Healthcare Providers
Sept. 15, 2009	Energy and Commerce	Preparing for the 2009 Pandemic Flu
Sept. 29, 2009	Oversight and Government Reform	The Administration's Flu Vaccine Program: Health, Safety, and Distribution

Table 2. (Continued)

Date	Committee (/Subcommittee)	Topic
Oct. 27, 2009	Homeland Security / Subcommittee on Emerging Threats, Cybersecurity and Science, and Technology	Real-Time Assessment of the Federal Response to Pandemic Influenza
Nov. 17, 2009	Education and Labor	Protecting Employees, Employers and the Public: H1N1 and Sick Leave Policies
Nov. 18, 2009	Energy and Commerce / joint Health, Oversight and Investigations	H1N1 Preparedness: An Overview of Vaccine Production and Distribution

Source: Compiled by Congressional Research Service.

Notes: Hearings were held in Washington, DC unless otherwise noted. A Member briefing was held by the House Appropriations Subcommittee on Labor, Health and Human Services, Education, and Related Agencies on November 4, 2009, with panelists from HHS, and from state and local health agencies.

a. Field hearing in Hartford, CT.

APPROPRIATIONS AND FUNDING

Public Health Emergency Funding Mechanisms

The Secretary of HHS does not have a dedicated source of funds to support the response to public health emergencies such as the current flu pandemic. Funds available to HHS from prior-year appropriations for pandemic flu could have supported vaccine development and modest procurements, but would not have been adequate for procurements and related activities sufficient to support a mass-vaccination campaign. GAO has noted that the *National Strategy for Pandemic Influenza: Implementation Plan* (2006), which lays out 324 action items for federal agencies to prepare for and respond to a flu pandemic, contains no discussion of the possible costs of these actions, or how they would be financed.[91]

Upon the determination of a public health emergency pursuant to Section 319 of the Public Health Service Act, the Secretary of HHS may access a no-year Public Health Emergency Fund. Such a determination was made with respect to the H1N1 flu outbreak on April 26. (See the earlier section "Determination of a Public Health Emergency.")[92] The fund has not received a recent appropriation and does not have a balance, however, so the Secretary is not currently able to use this funding mechanism for the pandemic response.

There has not been a Stafford Act declaration for the current flu pandemic, so disaster relief funds administered by the Federal Emergency Management Agency (FEMA) are not available for response efforts. Many relevant activities may not be eligible for Stafford funds, even if they were available.[93] (See the earlier section, "Applicability of the Stafford Act.")

The Secretary has authority to use a Covered Countermeasure Process Fund to compensate individuals for harm that results from their use of medical countermeasures, as identified in a declaration issued by the HHS Secretary.[94] A declaration was issued for the use of the antiviral drugs Tamiflu and Relenza for a possible pandemic flu virus in October 2008.[95] As noted earlier, a declaration was issued for the use of H1N1 pandemic vaccines in June, 2009.[96] Compensation could be provided for serious physical injuries or deaths resulting from the use of these products in this situation, including for unapproved uses pursuant to an Emergency Use Authorization. (See "FDA: Emergency Use Authorizations.") In FY2009 emergency supplemental funding for pandemic preparedness (P.L. 111-32), Congress authorized the use of an unspecified amount of the appropriation for the Covered Countermeasure Process Fund, and President Obama has sought to use contingent funds provided under the law for this purpose.[97]

Emergency Supplemental Appropriations for FY2009[98]

In June, the Obama Administration requested $2 billion in FY2009 emergency supplemental appropriations for response to the H1N1 threat, and authority to transfer additional amounts, totaling almost $7 billion, from existing HHS accounts. The Supplemental Appropriations Act, FY2009 (P.L. 111-32), signed on June 24, 2009, provided $1.9 billion in supplemental appropriations immediately,[99] and an additional $5.8 billion contingent upon a presidential request documenting the need for additional funds. Amounts provided are as follows:[100]

- $1.85 billion to the HHS Public Health and Social Services Emergency Fund (PHSSEF), available until expended, including not less than $200 million to CDC for several specified activities, and not less than $350 million for state and local public health response capacity.

- Of the $1.3 billion to HHS not specifically designated, the Secretary may transfer funds to other HHS accounts and to other federal agencies. Also, these funds may be used for purchases for the Strategic National Stockpile (SNS), for construction or renovation of privately owned vaccine production facilities, and for the Covered Countermeasure Process Fund (CCPF).
- An additional contingent emergency appropriation of $5.8 billion to the HHS PHSSEF would become available for obligation 15 days after the President provided a detailed written request to Congress to obligate specific amounts for specific purposes, and only if needed to address the emergency. If such requirements were met, funds could generally be made available and transferred as above, including for purchases for the SNS and the CCPF. However, contingent funds could not be used for construction or renovation of privately owned vaccine production facilities.
- $50 million to the President for the Global Health and Child Survival account to support global efforts to control the spread of the outbreak.
- The conference report provided that if WHO were to announce that the current outbreak had progressed to a flu pandemic (i.e., Phase 6),[101] and upon the President's determination and notification to Congress, available funds in four accounts from prior appropriations acts for the Department of State, Foreign Operations, and Related Programs—Global Health and Child Survival; Development Assistance; Economic Support Fund; and Millennium Challenge Corporation—may be used for pandemic response activities.

President Obama has twice requested portions of the contingent funding, totaling $4.541 billion, leaving a balance of $1.259 billion that the President may request at a later date. On July 16, the President requested $1.825 billion of the contingent appropriation, to be used for procurement of vaccine adjuvant, immunization campaign planning, FDA regulatory activities, and funding for the CCPF.[102] On September 2, the President requested an additional $2.716 billion of the contingent appropriation, to be used for the Departments of Agriculture, Defense, HHS, State, and Veterans Affairs to support the procurement of vaccine product and supplies, antiviral medications, preparations for a vaccination campaign, and agency preparedness activities.[103]

Prior Funding for Pandemic Flu Preparedness

In the fall of 2005, in the aftermath of Hurricane Katrina, and as H5N1 avian flu was spreading across several continents, Congress provided $6.1 billion in FY2006 supplemental appropriations for pandemic planning across several federal departments and agencies.[104] Since then, annual funding has been provided to CDC, FDA, and for other activities in HHS to continue work on vaccine development, stockpiling of countermeasures, and assistance to states. In total, from FY2004 through FY2009, HHS has received almost $13.4 billion for pandemic flu preparedness.[105] (See **Table 3**.) The U.S. Departments of Agriculture and the Interior have also received annual funding to monitor avian flu in domestic poultry and wild birds, respectively. The U.S. Agency for International Development (USAID) has received funds to assist other countries in managing avian flu transmission to humans, and preparing for a possible pandemic.[106]

In addition to amounts it specifically appropriates, Congress is also interested in how agencies budget for influenza within their existing activities. However, defining such amounts is difficult, for two reasons. First, for many years, domestic public health capacity for infectious disease control has moved away from "categorical" funding and programs (i.e., one disease at a time), and toward the development of flexible capacity that can adapt to new, unanticipated threats. These flexible surveillance systems, laboratory networks, communications platforms, and other capabilities can pivot rapidly to address new threats. But because pandemic planning efforts are tightly woven into the fabric of these flexible capabilities, it is not easy to tease out threads that describe the nation's investment solely for pandemic flu preparedness. Attempt to do so requires making judgments about what is "in" and "out" of scope that are somewhat arbitrary.

Second, for similar reasons, it can be difficult to tease apart investments made for pandemic flu, versus seasonal flu, versus avian or swine flu, versus investments in drug and vaccine development in general. Because different agencies use different methods and assumptions to account for their influenza spending, these amounts are not necessarily comparable between agencies, and caution is advised in adding such amounts together as if they were comparable.

HHS has tracked its pandemic influenza funding for the past several fiscal years, using comparable criteria from year to year. These amounts are presented in the department's annual budget requests, in sections designated for pandemic influenza, and are presented in **Table 3**.

Table 3. HHS Funding for Pandemic Influenza, FY2004-FY2010 (Dollars in Millions, Rounded)

Agency/ Activity	FY2004	FY2005	FY2006[a]	FY2007	FY2008	FY2009 regular[b]	FY2009 supp.[c]	FY2010 req.
OS and/or PHSSEF	50	99	5,152	0	75	585	6,391	354
CDC	0	0	400	70	155	156	0	156
FDA	0	0	20	33	35	39	0	39
NIH	0	0	18	35	34	35	0	35
TOTAL, Program Level	**50**	**99**	**5,590[d]**	**138**	**299**	**815**	**6,391[c]**	**584**

Source: Compiled by Congressional Research Service from HHS annual "Budget in Brief" documents at http://www.hhs.gov/asrt/ob/docbudget/, unless otherwise noted below.

Notes: OS is Office of the HHS Secretary. PHSSEF is Public Health and Social Services Emergency Fund, an account administered by the Secretary, which Congress has typically used to provide one-time funding for non-routine activities. NIH is the National Institutes of Health.

a. Appropriated in P.L. 109-148, the Department of Defense, Emergency Supplemental Appropriations to Address Hurricanes in the Gulf of Mexico, and Pandemic Influenza Act, 2006, and P.L. 109-234, the Emergency Supplemental Appropriations Act for Defense, the Global War on Terror, and Hurricane Recovery, 2006. Funds are available until expended.

b. Appropriated in P.L. 111-8, the Omnibus Appropriations Act, 2009. Pandemic flu funding was not included in P.L. 111-5, the American Recovery and Reinvestment Act of 2009 (ARRA).

c. Appropriated in P.L. 111-32, the Supplemental Appropriations Act, 2009. The Act provided the Secretary of HHS with $1.850 billion initially and an additional $5.8 billion contingent upon presidential request and demonstration of need. For more information, see CRS Report R40531, *FY2009 Spring Supplemental Appropriations for Overseas Contingency Operations*, coordinated by Stephen Daggett and Susan B. Epstein. Amount includes the initial amount (i.e., $1.850 billion) plus $4.541 billion in contingent appropriations. (President Obama requested $1.825 billion in contingent appropriations on July 16, and an additional $2.716 billion on September 2. See footnote 102 and footnote 103.)

d. Total does not include $30 million in supplemental funding to HHS that was transferred to the U.S. Agency for International Development (USAID).

U.S. PANDEMIC INFLUENZA PREPAREDNESS DOCUMENTS

In the George W. Bush Administration, pandemic flu preparedness efforts were coordinated by the Homeland Security Council.[107] Numerous federal and other documents that are specific to preparedness and response for a flu pandemic have been published. Selected documents are listed below. These plans are intended to address a pandemic caused by any so-designated flu strain, but they were written when there was significant global concern about H5N1 avian flu. To date, that flu strain has behaved quite differently from the H1N1 pandemic strain. In particular, the H5N1 strain has not shown the ability to transmit efficiently from person to person, but human infections that result directly from contact with infected poultry have generally been very severe, and there has been a high fatality rate.[108]

Unless otherwise noted, the U.S. pandemic flu plans below can be found on a government-wide pandemic flu website managed by HHS.[109]

- The *National Strategy for Pandemic Influenza,* November 2005, published by the Homeland Security Council, outlines general responsibilities of individuals, industry, state and local governments, and the federal government in preparing for and responding to a pandemic.
- *National Strategy for Pandemic Influenza, Implementation Plan,* May 2006, published by the Homeland Security Council, assigns more than 300 preparedness and response tasks to departments and agencies across the federal government; includes measures of progress and timelines for implementation; provides initial guidance for state, local, and tribal entities, businesses, schools and universities, communities, and non-governmental organizations on the development of institutional plans; provides initial preparedness guidance for individuals and families. One- and two-year implementation status reports have also been published.
- The *HHS Pandemic Influenza Plan,* November 2005, provides guidance to national, state and local policy makers and health departments, outlining key roles and responsibilities during a pandemic and specifying preparedness needs and opportunities. This plan emphasizes specific preparedness efforts in the public health and health care sectors.

- The *HHS Pandemic Influenza Implementation Plan, Part I,* November 2006, discusses department-wide activities: disease surveillance; public health interventions; medical response; vaccines, antiviral drugs, diagnostic tests, and personal protective equipment (PPE); communications; and state and local preparedness.
- *Interim Pre-pandemic Planning Guidance: Community Strategy for Pandemic Influenza Mitigation in the United States–Early Targeted Layered use of Non-Pharmaceutical Interventions,* February 2007, published by CDC, guidance for "social distancing" strategies to reduce contact between people, with respect to: closing schools; canceling public gatherings; planning for liberal work leave policies; teleworking strategies; voluntary isolation of cases; and voluntary quarantine of household contacts.
- *Department of Defense Implementation Plan for Pandemic Influenza,* August 2006, provides policy and guidance for the following priorities: (1) force health protection and readiness; (2) the continuity of essential functions and services; (3) Defense support to civil authorities (i.e., federal, state, and local governments); (4) effective communications; and (5) support to international partners.
- *VA Pandemic Influenza Plan*, March 2006, provides policy and instructions for Department of Veterans Affairs (VA) in protecting its staff and the veterans it serves, maintaining operations, cooperating with other organizations, and communicating with stakeholders.
- *Pandemic Influenza Preparedness, Response, and Recovery Guide for Critical Infrastructure and Key Resources*, published by DHS, September 2006, provides business planners with guidance to assure continuity during a pandemic for facilities comprising critical infrastructure sectors (e.g., energy and telecommunications) and key resources (e.g., dams and nuclear power plants).
- *State pandemic plans:* All states were required to develop and submit specific plans for pandemic flu preparedness, as a requirement of grants provided by HHS.[110]

KEY INFORMATION SOURCES

CRS Reports and Experts

2009 H1N1 "Swine Flu": CRS Experts: CRS Report R40845, *2009 H1N1 "Swine Flu": CRS Experts*, by Sarah A. Lister.

Current CRS Reports on public health and emergency preparedness in general:

http://apps.crs.gov/cli/cli.aspx?PRDS_CLI_ITEM_ID=3276&from=3&fromId=13

Current CRS Reports on specific aspects of the pandemic influenza threat:

- CRS Report R40560, *The 2009 Influenza Pandemic: Selected Legal Issues*, coordinated by Kathleen S. Swendiman and Nancy Lee Jones.
- CRS Report RS21414, *Mandatory Vaccinations: Precedent and Current Laws*, by Kathleen S. Swendiman.
- CRS Report RL34724, *Would an Influenza Pandemic Qualify as a Major Disaster Under the Stafford Act?* by Edward C. Liu.
- CRS Report R40531, *FY2009 Spring Supplemental Appropriations for Overseas Contingency Operations*, coordinated by Stephen Daggett and Susan B. Epstein.
- CRS Report R40575, *Potential Farm Sector Effects of 2009 H1N1 "Swine Flu": Questions and Answers*, by Renée Johnson.
- CRS Report R40588, *The 2009 Influenza Pandemic: U.S. Responses to Global Human Cases*, by Tiaji Salaam-Blyther.
- CRS Report R40619, *The Role of the Department of Defense During A Flu Pandemic*, by Lawrence Kapp and Don J. Jansen.
- CRS Report RL33609, *Quarantine and Isolation: Selected Legal Issues Relating to Employment*, by Nancy Lee Jones and Jon O. Shimabukuro.
- CRS Report RS21507, *Project BioShield: Purposes and Authorities*, by Frank Gottron.
- CRS Report R40570, *Immigration Policies and Issues on Health-Related Grounds for Exclusion*, by Chad C. Haddal and Ruth Ellen Wasem.

- CRS Report RL32724, *Mexico-U.S. Relations: Issues for Congress*, by Clare Ribando Seelke, Mark P. Sullivan, and June S. Beittel.
- CRS Report RL33381, *The Americans with Disabilities Act (ADA): Allocation of Scarce Medical Resources During a Pandemic*, by Nancy Lee Jones.
- CRS Report RS22327, *Pandemic Flu and Medical Biodefense Countermeasure Liability Limitation*, by Henry Cohen and Vanessa K. Burrows.
- CRS Report RL31873, *Banking and Financial Infrastructure Continuity: Pandemic Flu, Terrorism, and Other Challenges*, by N. Eric Weiss.
- CRS Report RS22264, *Federal Employees: Human Resources Management Flexibilities in Emergency Situations*, by Barbara L. Schwemle.

Archived CRS Reports on the threat of pandemic influenza: These products generally discuss concerns about a possible human flu pandemic resulting from H5N1 avian influenza, and enhanced federal preparedness efforts during 2005 through 2007.

- CRS Report RL33145, *Pandemic Influenza: Domestic Preparedness Efforts*, by Sarah A. Lister.
- CRS Report RL33219, *U.S. and International Responses to the Global Spread of Avian Flu: Issues for Congress*, by Tiaji Salaam-Blyther.
- CRS Report RS22576, *Pandemic Influenza: Appropriations for Public Health Preparedness and Response*, by Sarah A. Lister.

World Health Organization (WHO) Information

- Information about the current H1N1 pandemic flu situation: http://www.who.int/csr/ disease/swineflu/en/index.html (See also the **Appendix**.)
- Pandemic Influenza Preparedness and Response: A WHO Guidance Document, (April 2009): *http://www.who.int/csr/disease/influenza/pip* guidance2009/en/ index.html

- Current phase of flu pandemic alert: *http://www.who.int/csr/disease/ avian*nza/ phase/en/index.html
- Pan American Health Organization (PAHO), a regional office of the WHO, H1N1 flu page: *http://new.paho.org/hq/index.php?option=c* om_content&task=blogcategory& id=805&Itemid=569
- International Health Regulations (2005): http://www.who.int/topics/ international_health_regulations/en/

U.S. Federal Government Information

- Government-wide information: http://www.flu.gov/
- DHS, "Department Response to H1N1 (Swine) Flu," with links to information in other federal departments and agencies: *http://www.dhs* .gov/xprepresp/programs/ swine-flu.shtm
- CDC, H1N1 (swine flu) page: http://www.cdc.gov/h1n1flu/
- CDC Public Health Law Program, 2009 H1N1 Flu Legal Preparedness, http://www2a.cdc.gov/phlp/H1N1flu.asp
- FDA, 2009 H1N1 (Swine) Flu Virus, *http://www.fda.gov/NewsEv* ents/ PublicHealthFocus/ucm150305.htm
- Centers for Medicare and Medicaid Services (CMS), H1N1 information page, http://www.cms.hhs.gov/H1N1/
- U.S. Department of Education, H1N1 Flu Information, http://www.ed.gov/admins/ lead/safety/emergencyplan/pandemic/ ind ex.html
- U.S. Department of Agriculture (USDA), H1N1 Flu, http://www.usda.gov/wps/ portal/?navid=USDA_H1N1
- USDA nutrition program policies for pandemic flu, *http://www.fns.u* sda.gov/ disasters/pandemic/default.htm
- Department of Defense Pandemic Influenza Watchboard: http://fhp.osd.mil/ aiWatchboard/
- HHS Pandemic Planning Updates, addressing monitoring and surveillance, vaccines, antiviral medications, state and local preparedness, and communications, through January 2009: *http://www* .flu.gov/professional/federal/index.html (Note: much of this information is in the context of planning for the H5N1 avian flu threat.)

Additional Information

- Canada: Public Health Agency of Canada: http://www.phac-aspc.gc.ca/alert-alerte/ swine_200904-eng.php; Canadian Food Inspection Agency: *http://www.inspection.gc.ca/english/anim* a/disemala/swigri/swigrie.shtml
- Security and Prosperity Partnership of North America, *North American Plan for Avian and Pandemic Influenza,* August 2007, http://www.spp-psp.gc.ca/eic/site/spp-psp.nsf/vwapj/pandemic-influenza.pdf/$FILE/pandemic-influenza.pdf
- Center for Infectious Disease Research and Policy (CIDRAP), at the University of Minnesota, frequent updates, including scientific and technical information, *http://www.cidrap.umn.edu/cidrap/content/infl uenza*/swineflu/index.html
- Public Health Law and Policy Program at the Sandra Day O'Connor College of Law, at Arizona State University, Global Legal Triage and the 2009 H1N1 Outbreak (including prior and existing declared emergencies at the federal and state levels), *http://www.law* .asu.edu/?id=2036

Appendix. Key Official Actions by WHO

Determination of Influenza Pandemic Phase

The World Health Organization is the coordinating authority for health within the United Nations system. It is responsible for providing leadership, guiding a research agenda, setting norms and standards, articulating evidence-based policy options, providing technical support to countries, and monitoring and assessing health trends. WHO does not have enforcement powers.

An influenza pandemic occurs when a novel flu strain emerges and spreads across the globe, causing human illnesses. For that to happen, the virus must have the following features: it must be genetically novel so that there is a lack of preexisting immunity; it must be pathogenic (i.e., capable of causing illness in humans); and it must be easily transmitted from person to person.

Table A-1. WHO Influenza Pandemic Phases (Current Alert Level is Highlighted)

Phase	Description
Phase 1	No animal influenza virus circulating among animals has been reported to cause infection in humans.
Phase 2	An animal influenza virus circulating in domesticated or wild animals is known to have caused infection in humans and is therefore considered a specific potential pandemic threat.
Phase 3	An animal or human-animal influenza reassortant[a] virus has caused sporadic cases of small clusters of disease in people, but has not resulted in human-to-human transmission sufficient to sustain community-level outbreaks.
Phase 4	Human-to-human transmission of an animal or human-animal influenza reassortant[a] virus able to sustain community-level outbreaks has been verified.
Phase 5	The same identified virus has caused sustained community-level outbreaks in two or more countries in one WHO region.[b]
Phase 6	An influenza pandemic. In addition to the criteria defined in Phase 5, the same virus has caused sustained community-level outbreaks in at least one other country in another WHO region.[b]
Post-peak Period	Levels of pandemic influenza in most countries with adequate surveillance have dropped below peak levels.
Possible New Wave	Level of pandemic influenza activity in most countries with adequate surveillance rising again.
Post-pandemic Period	Levels of influenza activity have returned to the levels seen for seasonal influenza in most countries with adequate surveillance.

Source: Adapted by CRS from WHO, *Pandemic Influenza Preparedness and Response: A WHO Guidance Document*, April 2009, Table 1, p. 13, http://www.who.int/csr/disease/influenza/pipguidance2009/en/index.html.

a. A reassortant virus results from a genetic reassortment process in which genes from animal and human influenza viruses mix together to create a new strain.

b. WHO governs through six regional offices that do not strictly correspond with the world's continents. The WHO regions are the African Region; the Region of the Americas; the South-East Asia Region; the European Region; the Eastern Mediterranean Region; and the Western Pacific Region. See "WHO–Its People and Offices," http://www.who.int/about/structure/en/index.html.

WHO, in consultation with experts in member countries, monitors the spread of influenza among human populations, and has developed a scale to monitor pandemic risk. It consists of five "pre-pandemic" phases with increasing incidence of animal and then human illness and transmission, and a sixth phase that represents a full-blown human pandemic, with sustained viral transmission and outbreaks in most or all regions of the world. Historically, flu pandemics have occurred in multiple waves before subsiding. **Table A-1** describes the phases of a flu pandemic, as defined by WHO.

As a result of the rapid spread of the new flu strain, WHO raised the pandemic alert level from Phase 3, where it had been for several years because of the threat of H5N1 avian flu, to Phase 4 on April 27, and then to Phase 5 on April 29.[111] Phase 3 meant that a novel flu strain was causing sporadic small clusters of human illness, but was not sufficiently transmissible to sustain community-level outbreaks. Phase 4, by contrast, signaled that human-to-human transmission of the new H1N1 virus was sufficient to sustain community-level outbreaks. According to WHO, raising the alert level to Phase 5 meant that there was sustained community-level transmission in two or more countries within one WHO region, and that a pandemic could be imminent.

On June 11, WHO raised the level to Phase 6, declaring that an influenza pandemic, caused by the new H1N1 strain, was underway. According to WHO Director General Dr. Margaret Chan:

> Spread in several countries can no longer be traced to clearly-defined chains of human-to-human transmission. Further spread is considered inevitable.... The world is now at the start of the 2009 influenza pandemic. We are in the earliest days of the pandemic. The virus is spreading under a close and careful watch. No previous pandemic has been detected so early or watched so closely, in real-time, right at the very beginning. The world can now reap the benefits of investments, over the last five years, in pandemic preparedness.[112]

For several years, WHO urged governments, corporations, and other interests to develop pandemic influenza preparedness and response plans. Generally these plans are staged according to WHO pandemic phases. WHO has noted that under the current definitions, pandemic phases do not reflect the severity of illness, but rather the global extent of sustained community-level outbreaks. Some members of the public, however, had come to think of any flu pandemic as a catastrophic incident on the scale of the one that occurred in

1918, or that many feared could result from the deadly H5N1 avian flu if it became transmissible among humans. Some argued that the definition of a pandemic should be rewritten to take severity into account, and that a Phase 6 pandemic designation for the H1N1 flu situation would trigger over-reactions that were more disruptive than the disease.[113]

International Health Regulations

In 2005, the World Health Assembly adopted revised International Health Regulations (IHR), revising the roles and responsibilities of WHO and member states in the protection of international public health. The IHR(2005) require signatory nations (which include the United States) to notify WHO of all events that may constitute a "Public Health Emergency of International Concern," and to provide relevant information. The IHR(2005) also include provisions regarding designated national points of contact, definitions of core public health capacities, disease control measures such as quarantine and border controls (which are to be no more restrictive than necessary to achieve the desired level of health protection) and others.[114] On April 25, 2009, upon the advice of the Emergency Committee called under the rules of the IHR(2005), the WHO Director-General declared the H1N1 flu outbreak a Public Health Emergency of International Concern, thereby calling upon signatories to provide timely and transparent notification of events to WHO, to collaborate in disease reporting and control, and to adopt effective risk communication strategies to reduce the potential for international disease spread and the unilateral imposition of trade or travel restrictions by other countries.[115]

Travel Guidance

A number of governments have instituted enhanced passenger screening practices at their borders, and policymakers have debated more extensive prohibitions against the entry of travelers from countries or areas affected by the outbreak. The WHO has consistently advised against movement restrictions as a means to control influenza, citing a lack of evidence of their effectiveness, coupled with their potentially harmful effects on public confidence, local economies, and trade.[116]

Food Safety Guidance[117]

WHO has published a joint statement with Food and Agriculture Organization of the United Nations (FAO), the World Organization for Animal Health (known by its French acronym, OIE), and the World Trade Organization (WTO), saying:

> In light of the spread of influenza A(H1N1), and the rising concerns about the possibility of this virus being found in pigs and the safety of pork and pork products, we stress that pork and pork products, handled in accordance with good hygienic practices recommended by the WHO, FAO, Codex Alimentarius Commission and the OIE, will not be a source of infection.
>
> To date there is no evidence that the virus is transmitted by food. There is currently therefore no justification in the OIE Terrestrial Animal Health Standards Code for the imposition of trade measures on the importation of pigs or their products.[118]

End Notes

[1] See CRS Report RL33579, *The Public Health and Medical Response to Disasters: Federal Authority and Funding*, by Sarah A. Lister.

[2] See, for example, U.S. Government Accountability Office, *Influenza Pandemic: Gaps in Pandemic Planning and Preparedness Need to Be Addressed*, GAO-09-909T, July 29, 2009, pp. 6-7, http://www.gao.gov.

[3] Comments of DHS Deputy Secretary Jane Holl Lute, U.S. Congress, House Committee on Homeland Security, *Beyond Readiness: An Examination of the Current Status and Future Outlook of the National Response to Pandemic Influenza*, 111th Cong., 1st sess., July 29, 2009.

[4] Executive Office of the President, President's Council of Advisors on Science and Technology, *Report to the President on U.S. Preparations for 2009-H1N1 Influenza*, August 7, 2009, press release and link to full report at http://www.whitehouse.gov/ the_press_office/Presidents-Council-of-Advisors-on-Science-and-Technology-PCAST-releases-report-assessing-H1N1-preparations/ (hereafter referred to as PCAST report).

[5] This designation presumably refers to John Brennan, who serves as Assistant to the President for Homeland Security and Counterterrorism. For more information on the organization of the Homeland Security Council and its staff under the Obama Administration, see The White House, Office of the Press Secretary, "Statement by the President on the White House Organization for Homeland Security and Counterterrorism," press release, May 26, 2009, http://www.whitehouse.gov/briefing_room/PressReleases/.

[6] PCAST report, p. 32.

[7] The text of the President's Proclamation, "Declaration of a National Emergency with Respect to the 2009 H1N1 Influenza Pandemic," October 23, 2009, and related information are available at http://www.flu.gov/professional/ federal/h1n1emergency10242009.html. See also CRS Report 98-505, *National Emergency Powers*, by L. Elaine Halchin.

[8] Department of Homeland Security, *Remarks by Secretary Napolitano at Media Briefing on H1N1 Flu Outbreak*, April 27, 2009, http://www.dhs.gov/ynews/.

[9] CRS Report RL34758, *The National Response Framework: Overview and Possible Issues for Congress*, by Bruce R. Lindsay. The PFO position has been controversial, however, because it may conflict with the role of the Federal Coordinating Officer (FCO), a leadership position established in the Robert T. Stafford Disaster Relief and Emergency Assistance Act (the Stafford Act).

[10] CRS Report RL33053, *Federal Stafford Act Disaster Assistance: Presidential Declarations, Eligible Activities, and Funding*, by Keith Bea; and CRS Report RL33579, *The Public Health and Medical Response to Disasters: Federal Authority and Funding*, by Sarah A. Lister.

[11] CRS Report RL34724, *Would an Influenza Pandemic Qualify as a Major Disaster Under the Stafford Act?*, by Edward C. Liu.

[12] Homeland Security Council, *National Strategy for Pandemic Influenza: Implementation Plan*, May 2006, Appendix C, "Authorities and References," p. 212.

[13] FEMA, "Emergency Assistance for Human Influenza Pandemic," Disaster Assistance Policy 9523.17, March 31, 2007, at http://www.fema.gov/pdf/government/grant/pa/policy.pdf.

[14] Kevin Robillard, "Officials Say Swine Flu Vaccine is Coming," *CQ Homeland Security*, July 9, 2009.

[15] Comments of DHS Deputy Secretary Jane Holl Lute, U.S. Congress, House Committee on Homeland Security, *Beyond Readiness: An Examination of the Current Status and Future Outlook of the National Response to Pandemic Influenza*, 111th Cong., 1st sess., July 29, 2009.

[16] HHS, "October 24, 2009–President Obama Signs Emergency Declaration for H1N1 Flu," in particular the answer to the questions " ... How does the President's National Emergency declaration under the National Emergencies Act differ from a Stafford Act declaration? How does the request process for assistance under the Stafford Act differ from the request process for 1135 waivers?," *http://www.flu.gov/professional/federal/h1n1emergency10242009.html*.

[17] FEMA, "Disaster Assistance Fact Sheet 9580.106: Pandemic Influenza," October 22, 2009, http://www.fema.gov/ pdf/emergency/pandemic_influenza_fact_sheet.pdf.

[18] CDC, "Quarantine Stations," http://www.cdc.gov/ncidod/dq/quarantine_stations.htm.

[19] DHS, "Department Response to H1N1 (Swine) Flu," July 24, 2009, http://www.dhs.gov/files/programs/swine-flu.shtm.

[20] Donald G. McNeil, "Containing Flu Is Not Feasible, Specialists Say," *The New York Times*, April 29, 2009. See also WHO, *No Rationale for Travel Restrictions*, May 1, 2009, http://www.who.int/csr/disease/swineflu/guidance/ public_health/travel_advice/en/index.html.

[21] See "Closing the Border" in CRS Report R40560, *The 2009 Influenza Pandemic: Selected Legal Issues*, coordinated by Kathleen S. Swendiman and Nancy Lee Jones.

[22] See "Port of Entry Policies and Procedures" in CRS Report R40570, *Immigration Policies and Issues on Health-Related Grounds for Exclusion*, by Chad C. Haddal and Ruth Ellen Wasem.

[23] 42 U.S.C. § 247d. See HHS, "HHS Declares Public Health Emergency for Swine Flu," press release, April 26, 2009, http://www.hhs.gov/news. More information about this authority is available in CRS Report R40560, *The 2009 Influenza Pandemic: Selected Legal Issues*, coordinated by Kathleen S. Swendiman and Nancy Lee Jones; and CRS Report RL33579, *The Public Health and Medical Response to Disasters: Federal Authority and Funding*, by Sarah A. Lister.

[24] HHS, "Renewal of Determination that a Public Health Emergency Exists," July 24, 2009, http://www.flu.gov/ professional/federal/h1n1emergency072409.html; and October 1, 2009, http://www.flu.gov/professional/federal/ h1n1emergency100109.html.

[25] See "Section 1135 Waivers or Modifications" in CRS Report R40560, *The 2009 Influenza Pandemic: Selected Legal Issues*, coordinated by Kathleen S. Swendiman and Nancy Lee Jones.

[26] 42 U.S.C. § 1320b-5(b)(3). During a flu pandemic, patients can be relocated pursuant to a state's pandemic preparedness plan, if one exists. 42 U.S.C. § 1320b-5(b)(3)(B)(ii). For more information on EMTALA's requirements, see CRS Report RS22738, *EMTALA: Access to Emergency Medical Care*, by Edward C. Liu.

[27] 42 U.S.C. § 1320b-5(b)(7).

[28] The waivers and related information are available at CMS "H1N1 Overview," http://www.cms.hhs.gov/H1N1/.

[29] 42 U.S.C. § 1320b-5(b). When the 1135 waivers are available pursuant to a Stafford Act declaration, that declaration typically specifies the counties or other geographic areas in which emergency authorities are in effect. The determinations of both public health emergency and national emergency for the H1N1 pandemic apply nationwide.

[30] See CRS Report R40560, *The 2009 Influenza Pandemic: Selected Legal Issues*, coordinated by Kathleen S. Swendiman and Nancy Lee Jones. See also FDA, *Guidance: Emergency Use Authorization of Medical Products*, July 2007, *http://www.fda.gov/Regulatory* Information/Guidances/ucm125127.htm; and FDA/CDC, online course on Emergency Use Authorization, 2009, *http://www.bt.cdc*.gov/training/eua/index.html.

[31] Information is available at FDA, "Emergency Use Authorizations Questions and Answers," http://www.fda.gov/ NewsEvents/PublicHealthFocus/ucm153297.htm; and "Influenza (Flu) Antiviral Drugs and Related Information," *http://www.fda.gov/Dru* gs/DrugSafety/InformationbyDrugClass/ucm100228.htm.

[32] This approach should not affect medical care. Clinicians are advised to provide care, including treatment with antiviral drugs, based on the severity of a patient's symptoms, the presence of conditions that would place a patient at greater risk of severe infection, and other clinical considerations. It is not necessary that H1N1 flu be confirmed in order for appropriate treatment to be provided.

[33] CDC, "Reporting of Influenza and Pneumonia-Associated Hospitalizations and Deaths for the 2009-2010 Season," September 11, 2009, *http://www.cdc.gov/h1n1flu* /reportingqa.htm#surveillancesystems.

[34] CDC, "CDC Estimates of 2009 H1N1 Influenza Cases, Hospitalizations and Deaths in the United States, April – October 17, 2009," November 12, 2009, *http://www.cdc.gov/h1* n1flu/estimates_2009_h1n1.htm.

[35] Information in this section is drawn from CDC, "FluView," http://www.cdc.gov/flu/weekly/.

[36] See, for example, the figure by Sanofi Pasteur (a flu vaccine manufacturer), "A(H1N1) Vaccine Production Process," May 2009, *http://www.vaccineplace.com/d* ocs/H1N1productionprocess.pdf. A comparable figure showing the process for production of seasonal flu vaccine is at *http://www.vaccineplace.com/docs/Se* asonalfluproductionprocess.pdf. For additional information about flu vaccine development and manufacturing, see Congressional Budget Office, *U.S. Policy Regarding Pandemic-Influenza Vaccines*, September 2008, https://www.cbo.gov/ftpdocs/95xx/doc9573/09-15-PandemicFlu.pdf.

[37] For more information about the use of adjuvants, including safety concerns and possible effects on the global supply of pandemic flu vaccine, see Declan Butler, "Regulators Face Tough Flu-jab Choices," Nature News, July 21, 2009, *http://www.nature.com/new* s/2009/090721/full/460446a.html.

[38] See HHS, "HHS Takes Additional Steps Toward Development of Vaccine for the Novel Influenza A (H1N1)," press release, May 22, 2009; and HHS, "HHS Purchases Additional H1N1 Vaccine Ingredients," press release, July 13, 2009, (each at http://www.hhs.gov/news/). See, also, HHS, Biomedical Advanced Research and

Development Authority (BARDA), "H1N1 Vaccines," *http://www.hhs.gov /aspr/barda/index.html.*

[39] Information in this paragraph is drawn from NIH, National Institute of Allergy and Infectious Diseases (NIAID): "H1N1 Clinical Studies" at http://www3.niaid.nih.gov/topics/Flu/; and news releases at http://www3.niaid.nih.gov/ news/newsreleases/.

[40] FDA, "Vaccines Approved for H1N1 Influenza Virus," press release, September 15, 2009, http://www.fda.gov/ NewsEvents/Newsroom. See also FDA, "Influenza A (H1N1) 2009 Monovalent," which includes questions and answers and other information about all of the licensed pandemic vaccines, http://www.fda.gov/ BiologicsBloodVaccines/Vaccines/A pprovedProducts/ucm181950.htm.

[41] In the United States, seasonal flu vaccine is produced in multi-dose vials containing the preservative thimerosal, and in preservative-free single dose syringes. Thimerosal contains mercury. According to CDC, there is no convincing scientific evidence of harm caused by thimerosal in vaccines, but in 1999, the CDC, other federal agencies, the American Academy of Pediatrics, and vaccine manufacturers agreed that thimerosal should be reduced or eliminated in vaccines as a precautionary measure. As is the case for seasonal flu vaccine, a portion of the pandemic vaccine is being produced without preservatives for use in children and pregnant women. See CDC, "Mercury and Vaccines (Thimerosal)," http://www.cdc.gov/vaccinesafety/updates/thimerosal.htm.

[42] Information in this paragraph is drawn from CDC, "Questions and Answers on 2009 H1N1 Vaccine Financing," October 7, 2009, *http://www.cdc.gov/H1N1f* lu/vaccination/statelocal/vaccine_financing.htm.

[43] Unless otherwise noted, information in this paragraph is drawn from CDC, "H1N1 Flu Vaccination Resources," http://www.cdc.gov/h1n1flu/vaccination/.

[44] Robert Roos, "States to Designate Providers to Give H1N1 Vaccines," *CIDRAP News* (Center for Infectious Disease Research and Policy), August 10, 2009, *http://www.cidrap.umn.ed* u/cidrap/content/influenza/swineflu/news/ index.html.

[45] See for example testimony of Dr. Donald Williamson, Alabama Department of Public Health, and Mr. Rob Fulton, St. Paul Ramsey County, Minnesota, Department of Public Health, at a briefing of the House Appropriations Subcommittee on Labor, Health and Human Services, Education, and Related Agencies, November 4, 2009, http://appropriations.house.gov /Subcommittees/sub_lhhse.shtml.

[46] Comments of Dr. Jay Butler, Director of CDC's H1N1 Vaccine Task Force, transcript of CDC/FDA media briefing, August 21, 2009, http://www.cdc.gov/media/.

[47] Comments of Dr. Anne Schuchat, Director of CDC's National Center for Immunization and Respiratory Diseases, transcript of CDC media briefing, October 16, 2009, http://www.cdc.gov/media/. Although doses of the FluMist intranasal product were also available, that product could not be used in some of the prioritized high-risk groups such as pregnant women and those with chronic diseases.

[48] HHS, "2009 H1N1 Influenza Vaccine Supply Status," *http://www.flu.gov/indivi* dualfamily/vaccination/supply.html.

[49] Rebecca Ruiz, "Behind The H1N1 Vaccine Shortage," *Forbes*, October 30, 2009, and accompanying chart, "States With the Most and Least H1N1 Vaccine per 1,000 Residents," updated periodically.

[50] For information about public health recommendations for flu vaccination among health care workers, see CDC, "2009 H1N1 Vaccination Recommendations," *http://www.cdc.gov /h1n1flu/*vaccination/acip.htm. For information about the legal basis for mandatory vaccines, see CRS Report R40560, *The 2009 Influenza Pandemic: Selected Legal Issues*, coordinated by Kathleen S. Swendiman and Nancy Lee Jones; and CRS Report RS21414, *Mandatory Vaccinations: Precedent and Current Laws*, by Kathleen S. Swendiman.

[51] Unless otherwise noted, information in this paragraph is drawn from CDC, "H1N1 Flu Vaccination Resources," http://www.cdc.gov/h1n1flu/vaccination/.

[52] CDC, "Use of Influenza A (H1N1) 2009 Monovalent Vaccine: Recommendations of the Advisory Committee on Immunization Practices (ACIP), 2009," MMWR, vol. 58, August 21, 2009, http://www.cdc.gov/mmwr.

[53] Ibid.

[54] For a discussion of applicable state activities during the seasonal flu vaccine shortage of 2004-2005, see "Vaccine Rationing" in CRS Report RL32655, *Influenza Vaccine Shortages and Implications*, by Sarah A. Lister and Erin D. Williams.

[55] Unless otherwise noted, information in this section is drawn from CDC, "Vaccine Safety," http://www.cdc.gov/ h1n1flu/vaccination/vaccine_safety.htm.

[56] See http://vaers.hhs.gov/index.

[57] For more information, see Richard Neustadt and Harvey Fineberg, *The Swine Flu Affair: Decision-Making on a Slippery Disease* (U.S. Department of Health, Education, and Welfare, 1978), reprinted electronic edition at http://www.iom.edu/?id=65926.

[58] Department of Health and Human Services, Office of the Secretary, "Pandemic Influenza Vaccines–Amendment," *74 Federal Register* 30294-30297, June 25, 2009.

[59] For more information, see CRS Report RS22327, *Pandemic Flu and Medical Biodefense Countermeasure Liability Limitatio*n, by Henry Cohen and Vanessa K. Burrows, and "The Public Readiness and Emergency Preparedness Act (PREP Act)" in CRS Report R40560, *The 2009 Influenza Pandemic: Selected Legal Issues*, coordinated by Kathleen S. Swendiman and Nancy Lee Jones.

[60] In addition to liability waivers and compensation available for injuries related to the use of H1N1 pandemic vaccine, the PREP Act has also been invoked for the use of pandemic antiviral drugs, diagnostic tests, and protective equipment, as well as for the use of countermeasures for other threats such as anthrax and smallpox. See HRSA, "Countermeasures Injury Compensation Program: Covered Countermeasures," http://www.hrsa.gov/countermeasurescomp/ countermeasures.htm.

[61] Health Resources and Services Administration, "Preparedness Countermeasures Injury Compensation," http://www.hrsa.gov/countermeasurescomp/default.htm.

[62] H.Rept. 111-151, to accompany H.R. 2346, making supplemental appropriations for FY2009, June 12, 2009, pp. 114-115.

[63] The White House, Text of a Letter from the President to the Speaker of the House of Representatives, July 16, 2009, http://www.whitehouse.gov/the_press_office/Letter-from-the-President-regarding-H1N1/.

[64] Homeland Security Council, "National Strategy for Pandemic Influenza," November, 2005, p. 5, http://www.flu.gov/ professional/federal/index.html#national.

[65] HHS, "HHS Awards $487 Million Contract to Build First U.S. Manufacturing Facility for Cell-Based Influenza Vaccine," comments of Dr. Robin Robinson, Director of BARDA, press release, January 15, 2009, http://www.hhs.gov/news/.

[66] See for example PCAST Report, p. viii.

[67] The EMEA is responsible for the scientific evaluation of applications for authorization for medical products. Authorized products can be marketed in all European Union (EU) and EEA-EFTA states (Iceland, Liechtenstein and Norway). Product information is available at http://www.emea.europa.eu/.

[68] See comments of Anthony Fauci, Director, NIH National Institute of Allergy and Infectious Diseases (NIAID), House Appropriations Subcommittee on Labor, Health and Human Services, Education, and Related Agencies, "Briefing on Federal-State-Local H1N1 Flu Response," Nov. 4, 2009.

[69] Each of the approaches discussed here involve growing or replicating virus subunits in cells of one kind or another at some point in the process. These approaches are "cell-based" in that sense. However, when discussing technologies that are currently available for making flu vaccine, the term "cell-based" usually refers to the process for growing whole influenza virus, to distinguish it from the egg-based process.

[70] For more information on clinical trials, see NIH, "Understanding Clinical Trials," http://clinicaltrials.gov/ct2/info/ understand. FDA generally requires that Phase I through III clinical trials be conducted on medical products to demonstrate safety and effectiveness, in order for a product to be licensed.

[71] NIH, "Estimates of Funding for Various Research, Condition, and Disease Categories," http://report.nih.gov/rcdc/ categories/. The listing for influenza spending for FY2008 links to more than 300 funded projects.

[72] For more information about NIH research on influenza, see *http://www3.niaid.n* ih.gov/topics/Flu/; and "NIAID Influenza Research: 2009 Progress Report," http://www3.niaid.nih.gov/topics/Flu/PDF/fluResearch09.pdf.

[73] FY2009 emergency supplemental appropriations have been used for the immediate response to the H1N1 pandemic, including the development and procurement of H1N1 vaccine produced using eggs.

[74] The Sanofi Pasteur product is an injectable vaccine, produced in Swiftwater, PA. The Medimmune product is the intranasal vaccine, produced in Gaithersburg, MD.

[75] HHS, "HHS Awards $487 Million Contract to Build First U.S. Manufacturing Facility for Cell-Based Influenza Vaccine," press release, January 15, 2009, http://www.hhs.gov/news.

[76] HHS, BARDA, "Advanced Development of Recombinant Influenza Vaccine Products and Manufacturing Capabilities for Pandemic Preparedness," Solicitation Number HHS-BARDA-09-32, synopsis of presolicitation notice, April 17, 2009, http://www.fbo.gov. The solicitation was issued on July 10, 2009.

[77] See comments of Anthony Fauci, Director, NIH National Institute of Allergy and Infectious Diseases (NIAID), House Appropriations Subcommittee on Labor, Health and Human Services, Education, and Related Agencies, "Briefing on Federal-State-Local H1N1 Flu Response," Nov. 4, 2009.

[78] Funds are provided to the 50 states, DC, the territories, New York City, Chicago, and Los Angeles County.

[79] For more information, see the Appendix in CRS Report RL34190, *Pandemic Influenza: An Analysis of State Preparedness and Response Plans*, by Sarah A. Lister and Holly Stockdale; and CRS Report RS22576, *Pandemic Influenza: Appropriations for Public Health Preparedness and Response*, by Sarah A. Lister.

[80] Award amounts are available at HHS, "States Eligible to Receive $350 Million for H1N1, Seasonal Flu Preparedness Efforts," press release, July 10, 2009, http://www.hhs.gov/news/.

[81] CRS Report RL34190, *Pandemic Influenza: An Analysis of State Preparedness and Response Plans*, by Sarah A. Lister and Holly Stockdale.

[82] HHS and DHS, *Assessment of States' Operating Plans to Combat Pandemic Influenza: Report to Homeland Security Council*, January, 2009, *http://www.pandemicflu.gov/plan/st* ates/index.html. (Hereafter state assessment report).

[83] State assessment report, p. 43.

[84] See for example Rebecca Ruiz, "Behind The H1N1 Vaccine Shortage," *Forbes*, October 30, 2009, and accompanying chart, "States With the Most and Least H1N1 Vaccine per 1,000 Residents," updated periodically.

[85] For more information, see "School Closures" in CRS Report R40560, *The 2009 Influenza Pandemic: Selected Legal Issues*, coordinated by Kathleen S. Swendiman and Nancy Lee Jones, and CDC, "Guidance for Child Care Programs, Schools, Colleges and Universities," http://www.cdc.gov/h1n1flu/guidance/.

[86] James G. Hodge, Jr., Dhrubajyoti Bhattacharya, and Jennifer Gray, "Legal Preparedness for School Closures in Response to Pandemic Influenza and Other Emergencies," http://www.pandemicflu.gov/plan/school/ schoolclosures.pdf.

[87] CDC, "Change in CDC's School and Childcare Closure Guidance," press release, May 5, 2009, http://www.cdc.gov/ media/. See, also, U.S. Department of Education, "H1N1 Flu Information," http://www.ed.gov/admins/lead/safety/ emergencyplan/pandemic/index.html.

[88] CDC, "Update on School (K–12) and Child Care Programs: Interim CDC Guidance in Response to Human Infections with the Novel Influenza A (H1N1) Virus," May 5, 2009 (continually updated), http://www.cdc.gov/h1n1flu/ K12_dismissal.htm.

[89] HHS and DHS, *Assessment of States' Operating Plans to Combat Pandemic Influenza: Report to Homeland Security Council*, "Operating Objective B.4–Enhance State Plans to Enable Community Mitigation through Student Dismissal and School Closure," January 2009, pp. 25-26, http://www.pandemicflu.gov/plan/states/state_assessment.html.

[90] American College Health Association, "Pandemic Influenza Surveillance: Influenza Like Illness (ILI) in Colleges and Universities," http://www.acha.org/ILI_Surveillance.cfm.

[91] U.S. Government Accountability Office, *Influenza Pandemic: Continued Focus on the Nation's Planning and Preparedness Efforts Remains Essential*, GAO-09-760T, June 3, 2009, pp. 10-11, http://www.gao.gov. See also Homeland Security Council, *National Strategy for Pandemic Influenza: Implementation Plan*, May 2006, *http://www.pa* ndemicflu.gov/plan/federal/pandemic-influenza-implementation.pdf.

[92] For more information, see "Federal Funding to Support an ESF-8 Response," in CRS Report RL33579, *The Public Health and Medical Response to Disasters: Federal Authority and Funding*, by Sarah A. Lister.

[93] See "Federal Statutory Authorities for Disaster Response" and "Federal Funding to Support an ESF-8 Response," in CRS Report RL33579, *The Public Health and Medical Response to Disasters: Federal Authority and Funding*, by Sarah A. Lister. See also CRS Report RL34724, *Would an Influenza Pandemic Qualify as a Major Disaster Under the Stafford Act?*, by Edward C. Liu.

[94] CRS Report RS22327, *Pandemic Flu and Medical Biodefense Countermeasure Liability Limitation*, by Henry Cohen and Vanessa K. Burrows. The compensation program is administered by the Health Resources and Services Administration (HRSA) in HHS.

[95] HHS, "Declaration Under the Public Readiness and Emergency Preparedness Act" (notice regarding use of Tamiflu and Relenza), *73 Federal Register* 61861-61864, October 17, 2008.

[96] HHS, Office of the Secretary, "Pandemic Influenza Vaccines–Amendment," *74 Federal Register* 30294-30297, June 25, 2009.

[97] H.Rept. 111-151, to accompany H.R. 2346, making supplemental appropriations for FY2009, June 12, 2009, pp. 114-115.

[98] Information in this section is tracked in greater detail in CRS Report R40531, *FY2009 Spring Supplemental Appropriations for Overseas Contingency Operations*, coordinated by Stephen Daggett and Susan B. Epstein.

[99] Amount includes $1.85 billion to HHS for the Public Health and Social Services Emergency Fund and $50 million to the President for the Global Health and Child Survival account.

[100] H.Rept. 111-151, pp. 27-28, 34-35, 110, 114-116, 125-126, and 142.

[101] WHO declared the situation to be a flu pandemic, Phase 6, on June 11.

[102] The White House, Text of a Letter from the President to the Speaker of the House of Representatives, July 16, 2009, http://www.whitehouse.gov/omb/budget_amendments/.

[103] The White House, Text of a Letter from the President to the Speaker of the House of Representatives, September 2, 2009, *http://www.whitehouse.gov/omb/bud* get_amendments/.

[104] CRS Report RS22576, *Pandemic Influenza: Appropriations for Public Health Preparedness and Response*, by Sarah A. Lister.

[105] This amount includes funds made available through contingent transfer authority as provided in FY2009 supplemental appropriations, discussed in the previous section of this chapter. This amount excludes funds provided to other federal departments or agencies.

[106] Information can be found in CRS Reports on the applicable appropriations bills, at http://crs.gov/Pages/CLIs.aspx? CLIID=73, and: CRS Report R40239, *Centers for Disease Control and Prevention Global Health Programs: FY2001-FY2010*, by Tiaji Salaam-Blyther.

[107] Incident preparedness and response are different functions. At each level of government, they involve different leadership roles, legal authorities, organizational structures, and funding mechanisms. Generally, during an incident, certain conditions must be met before a jurisdiction can implement response activities, or access funds reserved for that purpose. With respect to the current H1N1 pandemic, the U.S. federal government has commenced pandemic flu response activities, under the overall coordination of the Secretary of Homeland Security.

[108] For more information about H5N1 avian flu and related public health concerns, see WHO, *Avian influenza*, http://www.who.int/csr/disease/avian_influenza/en/index.html; WHO, *Confirmed Human Cases of Avian Influenza A(H5N1)*, *http://www.who.int/csr/disea* se/avian_influenza/country/en/; and CRS Report RL33145, *Pandemic Influenza: Domestic Preparedness Efforts*, by Sarah A. Lister (archived).

[109] See http://www.flu.gov/professional/federal/index.html.

[110] For more information, see HHS, *Assessment of States' Operating Plans to Combat Pandemic Influenza: Report to Homeland Security Council*, January 2009, at http://www.pandemicflu. gov/plan/states/index.html, and CRS Report RL34190, *Pandemic Influenza: An Analysis of State Preparedness and Response Plans*, by Sarah A. Lister and Holly Stockdale.

[111] WHO, "Pandemic (H1N1) 2009," http://www.who.int/csr/disease/swineflu/en/index.html.

[112] WHO, "World Now at the Start of 2009 Influenza Pandemic" (Statement of Dr. Margaret Chan), press release, June 12, 2009, http://www.who.int/csr/disease/swineflu/en/index.html.

[113] See, for example, Robert Roos, "WHO Drawing Closer to Declaring a Pandemic," *CIDRAP News* (Center for Infectious Disease Research and Policy), June 2, 2009, http://www.cidrap.umn.edu/cidrap/content/influenza/swineflu/ index.html.

[114] For more information, see CRS Report R40560, *The 2009 Influenza Pandemic: Selected Legal Issues*, coordinated by Kathleen S. Swendiman and Nancy Lee Jones.

[115] WHO, *International Health Regulations*, http://www.who.int/ihr/en/. See, also, Rebecca Katz, "Use of Revised International Health Regulations during Influenza A (H1N1) *Epidemic,*" *Emerging Infectious Diseases*, vol. 15, no. 8 (August 2009), *http://www.cdc.gov/eid/content/15/8/1165.htm*.

[116] WHO, *No Rationale for Travel Restrictions*, May 1, 2009, http://www.who.int/ csr/disease/swineflu/guidance/public_health/travel_advice/en/ index.html.

[117] For more information, see CRS Report R40575, *Potential Farm Sector Effects of 2009 H1N1 "Swine Flu": Questions and Answers* , by Renée Johnson.

[118] *Joint FAO, OIE, WHO and WTO Statement on A(H1N1) virus*, May 2, 2009, http://www.wto.org/english/news_e/ news09_e/jt_stat_02may09_e.htm.

In: Influenza Pandemic: Response and Vaccine... ISBN: 978-1-61209-319-2
Editors: Adrian J. Buckman

Chapter 2

REPORT TO THE PRESIDENT ON REENGINEERING THE INFLUENZA VACCINE PRODUCTION ENTERPRISE TO MEET THE CHALLENGES OF PANDEMIC INFLUENZA*

Executive Office of the President

EXECUTIVE REPORT

Reengineering the Influenza Vaccine Production Enterprise to Meet the Challenges of Pandemic Influenza

Between April 2009 and February 2010, the United States experienced its most recent outbreak of pandemic influenza, this one resulting from the appearance of a novel strain ofType A, H1N1 virus. From the earliest recognition of the pandemic, public health officials in the United States moved rapidly to respond, but their efforts were impeded by unanticipated delays that arose in manufacturing what was supposed to be the most powerful tool for preventing widespread morbidity and mortality: a vaccine designed to protect against the 2009 H1N1 virus. Fortunately, the pathogenic potential of the 2009 H1N1 virus remained relatively mild, limiting morbidity and mortality,

* This is an edited, reformatted and augmented edition of an Executive Office of the President of the United States Report, dated August 2010.

although a disproportionate number of deaths occurred among children and young ad ults. This less-than-optimal experience—one that developed despite the appropriate and energetic response of vaccine manufacturers and public health officials—raised new awareness of the limitations of the system by which influenza vaccines are produced today.

At the request of the Executive Office of the President, the President's Council of Advisors on Science and Technology (PCAST) undertook a review of the processes currently employed for producing influenza vaccines. To execute this review, PCAST formed the Influenza Vaccinology Working Group, chaired by two of the PCAST co-chairs and further composed of six non-governmental experts in virology, immunology, vaccine manufacturing, and public health. PCAST considered ways the Federal Government might help to improve the technologies used for making vaccines for pandemic influenza, with a special focus on efforts that would address the following question:

How Can The Federal Government Help To Reduce The Time Required For The Nation To Supply Effective Vaccine To Its Population When The Next Influenza Pandemic Occurs?

It is useful to put this in a quantitative context by considering the time frame for action in 2009 and the future. In the case of 2009 H1 N1, the time between the declaration of a need for a vaccine against the pandemic virus and the start of the second wave of the pandemic in the United States was 18 weeks, and the time to the peak of the second wave was about 26 weeks. Each pandemic will surely differ, but this provides a reasonable indication of the time in which a large supply of effective vaccine might be required in subsequent pandemics.

The case of 2009 H1N1 also shows the challenges in meeting these time lines. Due to difficulties in producing vaccine, initial doses became available only after about 26 weeks, sufficient doses to cover half the population became available at 38 weeks and supply adequate to protect the entire Nation would have taken approximately 48 weeks to produce. This timeline was far too slow, by approximately 3 to 5 months.

Protecting the nation from an influenza pandemic thus requires tightening the schedule for making vaccine substantially: in a serious pandemic, saving weeks could translate into saving tens of thousands of lives.

With the goal of identifying ways to reduce the time to protect the public from the next pandemic, PCAST examined each step in the manufacturing process now used to make influenza vaccines, addressed the impact of improvements in each component on the time required to deliver the first doses of a new pandemic vaccine and to deliver all of the vaccine that would be required to protect the United States population. In addition, PCAST assessed a number of economic and regulatory issues that, regardless of technological developments, are potential barriers to improving the Nation's ability to protect its residents against pandemic influenza. In its review, PCAST also considered how changes in the production of pandemic influenza vaccines would affect the manufacture of seasonal influenza vaccines, and its work was also recognized as related to simultaneous studies of the larger United States medical countermeasure effort, which also includes vaccine development as part of its charge. PCAST's deliberations were informed by discussions with government officials and others in industry and academia with expertise in vaccine development and manufacturing.

In considering a path forward for reengineering the Nation's influenza vaccine enterprise, PCAST has developed a series of specific recommendations for action by the Federal Government. PCAST's analysis identified several components of the current influenza vaccine manufacturing process that could be improved substantially within the next two years without substantial alterations to the overall influenza vaccine enterprise, as well as transformations that will require action and support for the next two to six or more years. The effects of PCAST's recommendations on the delivery of pandemic influenza vaccines are summarized in Table ER-1 below. Comparisons of the approximate timelines for delivery of the first dose of vaccine are shown in Figure ER-1 for the current production method, using virus grown in embryonated chicken eggs, and for two of the most promising techniques for shortening those time lines, vaccines that uses viruses grown in cultured cells and those made with proteins produced with recombinant DNA technology.

PCAST has not determined anticipated costs for the projects required to make these improvements and has not attempted to allocate the share of financial responsibility to be borne by the governmental agencies or the companies. It is fair to assume, however, that an initial $1 billion in Federal funds—and at least similar sums over the subsequent few years—would be required to make the changes that will allow the Nation to mount a vigorous effort that can protect its population as well as possible in the event of another pandemic, an event that could have catastrophic consequences. Even in the relatively mild 2009 pandemic, over 2000 lives—mostly relatively young people, with an average age of less than forty—could have been saved if vaccination had begun even one month earlier. Furthermore, as this chapter makes clear, most of the Federal funds used to increase capacity to respond more quickly to influenza pandemics would also help to develop the technical platforms and production facilities that would support medical countermeasures more broadly against a variety of pathogens. For these reasons, an investment of $1 billion or more for several years can be justified on a cost:benefit basis.

Table ER-1. Effects of Recommended Actions on Delivery of Pandemic Influenza Vaccines

Recommended Change	Estimated Time Required to Make the Change	Effects on Time to First Dose	Effects on Bulk Production Until Demand Satisfied	Alternative Uses in Medical Countermeasure
Increased Surveillance	1-3 years	Moves the starting line forward by weeks or more	None	Yes
Faster Produc-tion of Optimal Vaccine Seed	1-2 years	Up to several weeks	Up to several weeks (if more efficient virus growth)	No
Modernized Sterility Tests	1-2 years	Approximately 1 week	None	Yes
Improved Generation of Potency Reagents	1-2 years	Avoids possible delay of up to several weeks	None	Possibly
Expanded and Streamlined Fill and Finish Procedures	1-3 years	Slight	Up to weeks	Yes
Shift to Cell Culture to make Killed Vaccine	1-3 years	A few weeks	Up to several weeks	Possibly
Shift to Cell Culture for Live Attenuated Vaccine	2-6 years	A few weeks	Up to several weeks	Possibly
Recombinant-based Vaccine	2-10 years	Several weeks	Up to several weeks	Yes

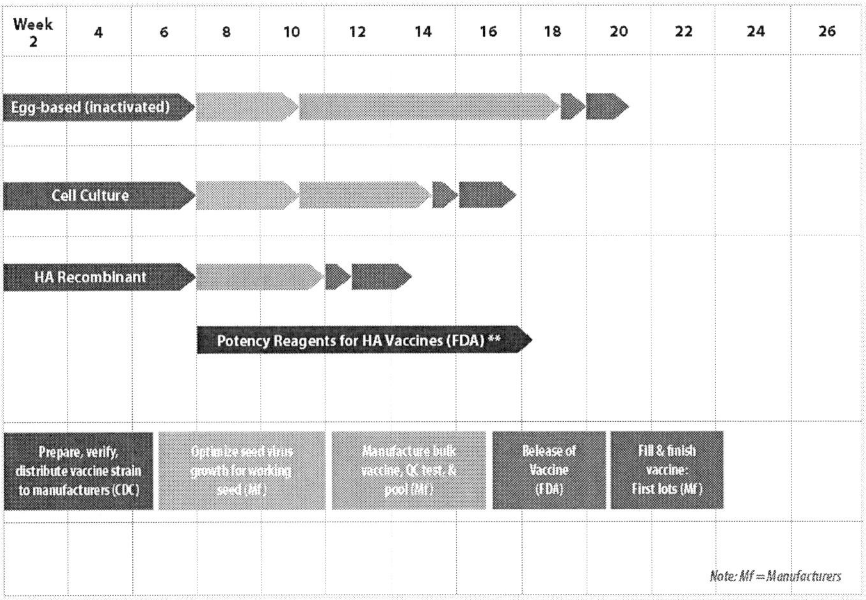

Approximate time lines to production of first dose of vaccine when producing inactivated influenza vaccine in chicken eggs and cell culture and recombinant vaccine produced in cell culture; time to final doses needed depends on manufacturing capacity.

Figure ER-1. A Comparison of Vaccine Production Timelines

Recommendations for Actions with Short-term Impact

Several recommended actions could improve the reliability and speed of delivering influenza vaccines over the next one to three years, without fundamental changes in the modes of manufacturing. Each of these actions could significantly shorten the time to delivery of the first doses of vaccine by one to several weeks. In the aggregate, these improvements could reduce the time predicted for first deliveries of vaccine after deciding to make a pandemic vaccine by approximately half of the current twenty weeks. Furthermore, improved surveillance could advance the start of the entire process of vaccine development by up to several weeks.

- **Accelerate the identification of new pandemic threats** by directing the Centers for Disease Control and Prevention (CDC) to fund the development and adoption of molecular platforms and supplement traditional clinical and microbiological methods that would enhance surveillance of human beings and certain animals for influenza viruses and other agents of respiratory illness.

Early detection of a viral pathogen, especially a pandemic strain of influenza virus, using the tools of modern molecular biology and diagnostic technologies can provide a powerful advantage by identifying a potential pathogen at an earlier time than is often possible with systems that are based largely on the recognition of overt disease in places thought to be at especially high risk. Earlier identification and reporting of the 2009 H1N1 virus could have helped to provide earlier delivery offirst doses and greater amounts of vaccine before the peak of the second wave of the pandemic by advancing the start of the vaccine production process.

- **Facilitate preparation of the virus strains to be used for vaccine production** (so-called"seed viruses") by directing the National Institute of Allergy and Infectious Diseases (NIAID) and the Biomedical Advanced Research and Development Authority (BARDA) to use focused contracts to ensure the development and dissemination of new influenza virus "backbones" that can exchange genes with new pandemic strains and are optimized for rapid growth.

  The difficulty of creating strains of influenza virus suitable for use as seed strains optimized to grow rapidly under the conditions used to manufacture influenza vaccine proved to be a major bottleneck in responding to the 2009 H1 N1 pandemic. Several technologically feasible options are available for hastening and regularizing the process of generating an initial seed strain. These include the development of a pre-existing set of viral backbones, increasing the likelihood that a highly proliferative seed virus can be quickly generated and that the initial seed virus will require little or no further optimization.
- **Shorten the time required for sterility testing of vaccines** (for influenza and other vaccines) before vaccine release, by directing BARDA and the Food and Drug Administration (FDA) to fund applied research that will adapt rapid nucleic acid amplification and sequencing methods to test for sterility, rather than depending on classical microbial assays.

  Each batch of vaccine material must pass a sterility test to ensure that it is not contaminated with bacteria or fungi. While current methods of doing this are reliable, they take approximately two weeks. More rapid sterility test methods, based on array-based sequencing methods and other technologies, are available and could cut the time for vaccine release by at least a week.

- **Shorten the time and increase reliability for preparation of reagents for potency testing,** by directing BARDA and the FDA to fund applied research that will develop rapid methods for assessing the concentration of antigenic materials, circumventing the need for production of new antibodies and/or traditional immunological tests.
  A critical step in manufacture of many vaccines, including inactivated influenza vaccines is testing vaccine material to determine the concentration of correctly folded antigen.This process is cal led "potency" testing, although it actually measures the amount of physical material that reacts with antibodies, rather than its true ability to induce an effective immune response.The method used today for testing potency of inactivated or killed vaccine is straightforward and by itself is not time consuming. However, the reagents used in the test are sheep antibodies raised against the viral protein hemagglutinin, and the steps required to produce those antibodies can take 8 to 12 weeks or longer if problems result. It should be possible, however, to develop new approaches to potency testing, using technologies available today that would eliminate the unpredictable nature of the current methods.
- **Assemble a manufacturing network with sufficient capacity** to rapidly fill the vials, syringes, and sprayers required for delivery of vaccines for influenza and other viruses, by working with industry to adopt advanced manufacturing practices, modify existing facilities, or construct new facilities. As part of this effort, the Federal Government, working closely with manufacturers, should undertake a comprehensive study within six months to quantitatively assess current fill-finish capacity and to develop a plan to ensure adequate capacity to produce sufficient quantities of pre-filled syringes, vials and/or nasal sprayers to meet the national need.

All vaccines must eventually be packaged.The"fill-finish"step for inactivated influenza vaccines involves transferring bulk vaccine into individual single-dose syringes as well as the single or multi-dose vials used for inactivated influenza vaccines or to nasal sprayers required for the live attenuated virus vaccines.This step is a major hurdle on the path to vaccine distribution to providers, and represents a costly and laborious phase of manufacturing that can be expanded only in a linear fashion, and it generally proves to be a major rate-limiting step in the process of delivering vaccine, especially under pandemic conditions.

Recommendations for Actions with Longer-Term Impact

In addition to examining the vaccine manufacturing enterprise with an eye on short-term fixes, PCAST also considered the prospects for making substantial changes in the composition of influenza vaccines or in the methods by which influenza vaccines are prod uced. These actions are likely to require significant additional investments on the part of both the Federal Government and the private sector, and they will require close collaboration between the private and public sectors. PCAST's recommendations for action that would substantially reengi neer the vaccine manufacturing enterprise over a longer time period include:

- **Understand current capacity for cell culture production and develop incentives to expand capacity.**
  PCAST recognized that without replacing the inherently time-consuming egg-based method of production with either a cell culture-based method or a recombinant DNA-based method of production, delivery of all of the needed vaccine, up to the last dose, will remain a long and unpredictable process. However, it is likely that existing facilities available for cell culture production do not have adequate capacity to meet vaccine demand. DHHS, DHS, and BARDA should lead a systematic, rapid study, involving governmental and non-governmental experts, of the requirements for and cost-benefit ratio of additional investments in cell culture manufacturing facilities. This study should also balance the magnitude of investment and time frame for expansion of cell culture facilities against the likelihood of developing approved recombinant influenza vaccines in the foreseeable future, the probability of another pandemic, and the advantages of greater use of live attenuated influenza vaccines.
- **Accelerate clinical research studies and regulatory approval for wider use of live attenuated influenza virus (LAIV) vaccines.**
  Influenza vaccines made with live attenuated influenza virus may be able to trigger a more effective immune response than can inactivate virus vaccines. As a result, production capacity demands in the event

of a pandemic would be lower if the majority of vaccine production was devoted to LAIV vaccines. However, the immunological basis of the clinical protection afforded by LAIV vaccines is not fully understood. Therefore, the FDA requires that LAIV vaccines—whether produced in chicken eggs or cell culture, be shown through an extensive efficacy trial to be as effective as inactivated virus vaccines currently produced in embryonated chicken eggs; the cost of such studies typically range from $50 million to as much as $100 mil lion. This cost is a major barrier to the more widespread development of LAIV vaccines, whether for seasonal or pandemic influenza.

- **Launch an aggressive initiative that supports the development, clinical testing, and approval of influenza vaccines made using recombinant DNA technology,** with the goal of achieving proofs-of-principle for at least three strategies for recombinant vaccines within three years.

  Recombinant DNA technology is already used to make vaccines against hepatitis B and human papilloma viruses, and early evidence suggests that recombinant DNA technology can also be used to create influenza vaccines. Using recombinant DNA technology and other advanced methodologies to produce influenza vaccines would shorten the time to both first and last dose of vaccine, and could offer other advantages for vaccine manufacturers.
- **Develop an investment strategy that allows flexibility in financing of promising vaccine production platforms, and create down-stream incentives for products that meet the target product profile and production criteria.**

  Given the commodity nature of the influenza vaccine market, it may be necessary for the Federal Government to establish downstream incentives, such as guaranteed purchases or a high-value prize, and to work in concert with venture capital firms and other investors to make direct investments in companies with promising next-generation vaccine platforms.
- **Support clinical tests of existing and new vaccines in the presence of adjuvants**, the development of a regulatory guidance document for adjuvants, and further research and development on adjuvants.

  By stretching the limited vaccine supply, addition of adjuvants to a vaccine formulation can shorten the time between provision of the first and last doses by several weeks. Adjuvants may also be required to elicit maximum immunity from vaccines produced using recombinant DNA technology.

- **Support basic immunology research aimed at understanding how the immune system responds to influenza virus** with the goal of developing a "universal" influenza vaccine that would provide broad protection for multiple years against both existing and new strains of influenza virus.

  Unlike most vaccines that afford long-term protection against pathogenic viruses, new influenza vaccines must be developed each time a novel influenza virus appears in the human population. However, recent research suggests that it may be possible to create a "universal"influenza vaccine that could provide broader protection against both seasonal and pandemic influenza, but additional work is needed to further explore the promise of developing such a vaccine.
- **Implement a new management structure for overseeing the mission-driven enterprise** to reengineer the Nation's influenza vaccine development and production enterprise.

  PCAST also recommends that the Administration develop a new management structure that vests authority with the Assistant Secretary for Preparedness Response (ASPR) at the Department of Health and Human Services (HHS) to coordinate and task component agencies at HHS with activities necessary to support the reengineering process recommended above. To assist with these activities, HHS should also establish a small advisory committee, comprised of representatives from the biotechnology, pharmaceutical and investment communities, to guide its engagement with industry. This committee's advice should be considered seriously in all decisions and actions by the Department, given the paramount importance of the relationship between the Federal Government and industry partners. Finally, all of the Administration's efforts to improve the Nation's capacity to respond quickly and effectively to the next influenza pandemic should be closely monitored by the White House, especially by the staff of the National Security Council.

I. INTRODUCTION, CHARGE, AND SUMMARY OF FINDINGS

SECTION SUMMARY

This introductory chapter describes the pandemic caused by a novel H1N1 strain of influenza virus in 2009; the difficulties in delivering vaccine to protect the US population against the second wave of the pandemic; and the convening of a Working Group, under PCAST, to study current methods for making vaccines against pandemic influenza, to recommend improvements in those methods, and to identify roles for the Federal Government in making those improvements. The chapter also outlines the nature of the relatively short-term and longer-term improvements that the Working Group has recommended in later chapters, and it describes both the components of the analysis (science, technology, public health, economics, regulation) and the relationship of the study to broader efforts by the United States to improve medical counter-measures against biological threats.

The Pandemic of 2009 and the Vaccine Problem

The 2009 influenza pandemic, caused by a novel strain of Type A, H1N1 virus (2009 H1N1), was initially detected as an unexpected outbreak of influenza-like illnesses in Mexico in mid-March, 2009. The virus spread rapidly in Mexico, the United States, and elsewhere; by June 11, the World Health Organization (WHO) declared a Phase 6 epidemic. (A more detailed summary of the 2009 pandemic is provided in Box 1-1 at the end of this chapter.)

From the earliest recognition of the pandemic, public health officials in the United States moved rapidly to respond. It was assumed that vaccines would be an essential countermeasure, likely the most critical, on a list that also included antiviral drugs, social measures to diminish transmission, and intensive care for the critically ill[1]. Ideally, vaccine would have been available before the second wave of the pandemic, which was expected to begin as early as late August. Yet when the second wave arrived, on schedule, the first doses of vaccine against the new strain of influenza virus were not available; in fact, they did not become available for use in the United States until October 5, about six weeks later. Moreover, only 124 million doses, enough to immunize about forty percent of United States residents, were distributed by the end of January, three months after the incidence of infection peaked in late October. As of April, 2010, an estimated 81-91 million doses of vaccine had been administered, covering about one-quarter of the US population. Much of it has still not been used, and little has been delivered to countries in the developing world. (A chronological account of vaccine production and delivery is also included in Box 1-2.)

Fortunately, the pathogenic potential of the 2009 H1N1 virus has remained relatively mild.The Centers for Disease Control and Prevention (CDC) estimates that 15 to 25% of the United States population was infected; between April 2009 and February 2010, 8500 to 17600 deaths were related to the pandemic. If this virus had been as lethal as those encountered in the more severe epidemics of the 20th century, the number of deaths in an unprotected United States population could have been 10- to 100-fold higher. Still, in contrast to the usual behavior of seasonal influenza, the burden of disease fell largely on young age groups: about 90% of hospitalizations and deaths occurred among people under the age of 65, and a disproportionate number of deaths (estimated by the CDC to be about 1280) occurred among those in the 0 to 17 year old age group.

While vaccine production fell short of the desired timetable, vaccine manufacturers and public health agencies operated appropriately and energetically, despite difficult circumstances. Vaccine makers typically produce seasonal influenza vaccine over a 9-10 month time frame that begins with the identification of viral strains by health officials in February and vaccine delivery in November or December of the same year. In contrast, the vaccine for the 2009 H1N1 virus was prepared and the initial doses were distributed less than six months after identification of the virus. Even so, that was too late to provide protection for most of the United States population, since the second wave of the pandemic began in the United States in late August and distribution of the bulk of the vaccine did not occur for another three or four months. (A brief description of the properties of influenza viruses responsible for seasonal and pandemic influenza and of the corresponding vaccines can be found in Box 1-3.)

As will be described in detail in Chapter 2, the time to delivery of vaccine against the 2009 H1N1 virus could have been considerably shorter if the virus had been detected and isolated earlier (allowing more time between isolation of the virus and the return of the pandemic), if the working seed virus for making vaccine had been more quickly optimized, and if the seed strains had grown more abundantly in eggs (allowing more efficient production of vaccine). In short, despite valiant efforts by Federal agencies and several commercial manufacturers, vaccine was not available to protect a large segment of the public against a potentially devastating infection.The fault lay not in the execution, but in the inherent shortcomings of current technologies for the development and production of influenza vaccines.

PCAST on Influenza Vaccinology and its Charge

This sobering experience with 2009 H1N1 vaccines has refocused attention on national preparedness against infectious agents in general and against influenza viruses in particular. In August of 2009, before the second wave of the pandemic occurred in the United States, the President's Council of Advisors on Science and Technology (PCAST) published a report on the various measures that were being taken to combat the on-going pandemic.[2] While praising those efforts, the report also cautioned that vaccine was unlikely to arrive in time to protect the most vulnerable people—those who would normally receive the first doses of vaccine—and that production might also be inadequate to protect the majority of all people before the second wave of the pandemic peaked.

When the pandemic subsided at the start of 2010, the Executive Office of the President (EOP) asked PCAST to revisit the processes currently employed for production of influenza vaccines, especially against pandemic influenza, and to consider whether and how the government might encourage the application of improved technologies to the problem of making influenza vaccines. In January 2010, PCAST formed a Working Group on Influenza Vaccinology, composed of experts in virology, immunology, vaccine manufacturing, and public health, to answer the following question:

How can the Federal Government help to reduce the time required for the nation to supply effective vaccine to its population when the next influenza pandemic occurs?

It is useful to put this in a quantitative context:

- The interval between the recognition in late April 2009 of the need for a vaccine and the start of the second wave of infection in late-August 2009 was about 18 weeks; in future pandemics, the interval could be shorter. The time to the peak of the second wave was about 26 weeks.

- The WHO's standard schedule for producing vaccine against pandemic influenza anticipates an approximately 20-week time schedule for initial availability of a new vaccine, with the subsequent time to produce enough doses to cover the entire nation depending on manufacturing capacity.
- In the case of 2009 H1N1, difficulties in producing a vaccine stretched this timeline: it was about 26 weeks until initial doses became available, it took a total of 38 weeks until sufficient supply was on hand to cover half the population, and it would have taken 48 weeks to have supply adequate to protect the entire Nation. This timeline was far too slow, by approximately 3 to 5 months.
- The timelines above focus only on vaccine production. Some additional time is required for vaccine distribution and administration, as well as 1-2 weeks for vaccinated individuals to gain immunity.

Protecting the nation from an influenza pandemic thus requires tightening the time schedule for vaccine production substantially. In a serious pandemic, saving weeks could translate into saving tens of thousands of lives.

To identify ways in which the time line could be shortened, PCAST considered: (i) each step in the WHO's schedule for producing vaccine against pandemic influenza; (ii) the events that determined the dates of delivery of vaccine during the 2009 H1N1 influenza pandemic; (iii) a wide range of options for shortening the time to delivery of vaccines (by altering the type of vaccine, the mode of production, and the steps required to develop a new vaccine in response to a pandemic); and (iv) the economic and regulatory issues that pose potential barriers to altered methodologies. PCAST then developed a set of recommendations to guide the Federal Government's efforts to improve the situation.

In addressing its question, PCAST took into account two aspects of the problem: the time to deliver initial supplies of vaccine ("time to first dose"), an important measure of protection of the most vulnerable, high-risk populations; and the time to deliver sufficient vaccine to meet the entire national need ("time to last dose"). The results of this analysis and PCAST's recommendations are described in detail in subsequent chapters.

The Analysis of the Problem and Major Findings

PCAST first reviewed all of the steps in the existing process that precede the packaging of finished vaccine products at manufacturing sites, with the intention of identifying procedures that could be improved or accelerated, assuming the country continues to depend on egg-based production of vacci nes. These steps include: the surveillance that detects and isolates viral pathogens; the generation of derivative viruses that can be used for vaccine production ("seed"viruses); the growth of virus in chicken eggs; the production of reagents for testing vaccine preparations for potency; sterility tests of the vaccine; and filling syringes, vials, or sprayers for delivery of the vaccine to the public. Events that follow the completion of manufacture—such as distribution of vaccine, prioritization of users, and administration by health care workers—are, of course, also important in management of a pandemic response, but were considered to lie beyond the group's charge and were not examined in detail.

PCAST then considered the prospects for making substantial changes in the composition of influenza vaccines or in the methods by which influenza vaccines are produced. In particular, it evaluated the relative merits of:

- continuing egg-based production of the two currently approved forms of influenza vaccines, chemically inactivated virus ("killed virus" vaccine) and live attenuated influenza virus (LAIV) vaccine;
- shifting to cell culture-based methods of virus production for these two vaccines;
- increasing the proportion of LAIV vaccine relative to killed virus vaccines;
- replacing vaccines composed of LAIV or killed virus preparations with the protein products of recombinant DNA technologies ("recombinant vaccines");
- adding immunological stimulants (adjuvants) to the killed vaccine preparation; and
- pursuing research to develop a "'universal" influenza vaccine that might provide protection against a wide range of influenza strains.

PCAST's analysis identified several components of current methodology that could be improved substantially even without altering fundamental vaccine production strategies.These findings and the recommended actions to be taken by the United States Government are described in detail in Chapter 3, along with the anticipated effects of the proposed improvements on the time required to provide the first doses of vaccine and to fulfill the goal of supplying enough vaccine to protect the United States population by vaccinating most or all of its residents. (Eighty percent of the population—requiring about 250 million doses of vaccine—is a realistic estimate of the vaccine recipients necessary to provide the optimal achievable protection.)

These relatively **short-term improvements,** potentially achievable in the next one to three years, include:

1. Increasing the time available for making vaccine after identification of a new pandemic strain by improving methods for **surveillance** for new respiratory viruses, including influenza viruses.
2. Shortening the time to provide the first dose of vaccine by streamlining the methodology for **producing the seed virus** (a virus strain that grows efficiently and carries the relevant immune components); for making reagents necessary for **potency tests;** for testing the **sterility** of vaccine preparations; and for placing vaccine materials in appropriate delivery devices ("**fill and finish**").
3. Insuring that vaccine is made available to people rapidly in an appropriately prioritized fashion.

Successful development and deployment of the recommended changes in production of egg-based vaccines could reduce the time to delivery of first doses of vaccine after identification of a new strain by as much as six to ten weeks of the 20 weeks currently envisioned by the WHO in the standard time line. In addition, better surveillance could advance the starting point for vaccine development, and streamlined delivery would get the first doses of vaccine to the appropriate target populations in a more timely manner.

PCAST recognized that, without replacement of the inherently time-consuming egg-based method of production, delivery of all of the needed vaccine, up to the last dose, will remain a long and unpredictable process. For that reason, PCAST also outlined paths towards more efficient vaccine production, based on several alternative methods, including production of virus in cell culture (Chapter 4), development of vaccines made with recombinant DNA technology (Chapter 5), and (in the more distant future) improved design of antigens to create a so-called universal vaccine that would elicit more durable and more cross-reactive immunological responses (Chapter 7).

Since it is difficult to predict how many years would be required for an effective recombinant vaccine to be approved and ready for wide-spread use, PCAST also considered increasing the proportion of LAIV vaccine, as opposed to killed virus vaccine, used to immunize against either pandemic or seasonal influenza. By combining the higher yield of LAIV vaccine with the more efficient cell culture-based production methods, significant savings could be made in time to delivery of last doses. But the shift to cell culture-based production of vaccine would also require new facilities, with economic consequences that need to be weighed with respect to the likelihood of another influenza pandemic and the alternative uses of cell culture facilities. This dilemma is discussed at greater length in Chapter 4.

PCAST also reviewed the potential utility of adjuvants in most of the contemplated vaccine strategies: egg-based, inactivated virus vaccines (in which adjuvants are known to increase effectiveness and are approved for use in Europe), cell-based inactivated virus vaccines (predicted to behave like egg-based vaccines of the same type), recombinant vaccines (which may **require** adjuvants, especially if they are composed of only a single viral protein), and universal vaccines. These issues are considered in depth in Chapter 6.

PCAST notes that while the urgent national need is to ensure protection against a severe pandemic, improvements will likely be implemented first in the context of annual production of vaccine against seasonal influenza. The reasons for this are obvious: seasonal influenza is a predictably recurrent, large-scale phenomenon, whereas pandemics are infrequent and difficult to anticipate; furthermore, seasonal and pandemic influenza vaccines are currently produced in an identical manner, with the vaccines differing only with respect to viral strains. (Indeed, the seasonal influenza vaccine for 2010 will incorporate the 2009-H1N1 strain.)

PCAST therefore considered in Chapter 2 the economics of seasonal influenza vaccine from the perspective of manufacturers. Influenza vaccine is a commodity product characterized by relatively low profit margins that fail to attract large investments to improve manufacturing processes. Notably, the WHO timeline for pandemic vaccine production is generally more than adequate for producing seasonal influenza vaccines in advance of annual winter outbreaks. Fundamental changes in the production methods used in such an industry will typically occur only slowly, especially since most of the newer methods still require further development, laboratory and clinical tests, and regulatory approval. PCAST thus discussed ways to create economic incentives to speed innovation.

Finally, PCAST has viewed this study as part of a wider effort to re-evaluate the nation's capacity to respond to various kinds of threats, including biological agents that emerge and re-emerge naturally or that serve as agents of bioterrorism. Influenza differs in many ways from certain biological threats, such as smallpox, anthrax, or other rare and often highly lethal agents, because of its regular (seasonal) recurrence on a large scale, the requirement for frequent vaccination, the need for large-scale dedicated production facilities for seasonal vaccines, and the virtual certainty of repeated pandemics, even though they cannot be accurately predicted. (See Box 1-3 on influenza viruses for an explanation of some of these phenomena.)

In his 2010 State of the Union Address, the President underscored the Administration's commitment to developing better medical counter measures against biological agents:

We are launching a new initiative that will give us the capacity to respond faster and more effectively to bioterrorism or an infectious disease—a plan that will counter threats at home and strengthen public health abroad.[3]

In response to the President's declaration, the Administration has undertaken a broader survey of countermeasures and the opportunities for improving them. While recognizing that influenza represents only one type of threat and that all threats have particular properties that must be appropriately considered, PCAST also believes that the scientific, technical, and economic challenges posed by influenza vaccinology are relevant to efforts to address other threats through, for example, the enhancement of surveillance, construction of shared technology platforms, improvements in regulatory science, and identification of economic incentives for industry.

1-1. Important Milestones in the 2009 Pandemic

- The first cases of what became the 2009 influenza pandemic were initially detected as influenza-like-illnesses in Mexico in late February and March.The first laboratory confirmed case, documented retrospectively, occurred on February 24, 2009.
- The novel type A influenza virus, referred to here as 2009-H1N1, was first identified by the CDC on April 15 in a respiratory specimen obtained from a child in California on April 1.The genome of this isolate was sequenced and designated A/California/05/2009(H1N1).

Specimens from two other cases, obtained on March 28 and March 30, were later confirmed to be H N1; these were the earliest documented H1N1 cases in the United States.

- Spread of H1N1 virus was quickly documented in many states in the United States and in other countries when the sequence of the virus was reported and specific testing could be done. Testing showed that the occurrence of influenza-like illnesses beyond the usual seasonal influenza epidemic period was usually caused by H1N1.
- The WHO determined that the spread of the new virus had been sufficient to declare a Phase 6 pandemic on June 11.
- While the number of cases declined in the Northern Hemisphere during the summer months, many cases were observed in the Southern Hemisphere, as was well-documented, for example, in Australia and New Zealand.The pandemic then resurged in late August in North America and Europe. The peak number of reported cases in the United States occurred in the last week of October, 2009.
- The pandemic is estimated by the CDC to have caused infection in 15 to 25% of the United States population, with between 8,520 and 17,620 2009 H1N1-related deaths between April 2009 and February 13, 2010.

1-2. Events Affecting Production of 2009 H1N1 Vaccines[4]

1. **Prepare, verify, distribute vaccine seed strain to manufacturers.** On April 27, the WHO recommended the use of the influenza A/California/05/2009(H1 N1) virus for vaccine production.This strain was isolated, prepared, and validated by the CDC, then a seed strain was prepared by reassortment with standard vaccine stocks.The CDC shipped this starting seed strain to manufacturers on May 26, 2009.
2. **Optimize seed virus growth.** In June, manufacturers tested the seed strain provided by the CDC and found that virus growth in eggs was not optimal for large-scale vaccine production. Manufacturers then used genetic methods to improve the working seed and were ready to begin bulk production between June 20-30, 2009.
3. **Manufacture bulk vaccine, QC test, & pool.** On July 16, the FDA notified manufacturers that the 2009 H1 N1 virus would be subjected to the release criteria normally used for seasonal vaccine, so the testing

was confined to measurement of "potency" (to assure that doses of inactivated virus vaccine contained 15 micrograms of hemagglutinin (HA) antigen) or to assay of infectious virus for LAIV vaccine. Clinical tests for induction of antibodies (with a hemagglutination inhibition [HAI] assay) were not required, although the inactivated vaccine was reported in early September to have the expected immunogenic potential as a single 15 microgram dose.The first bulk 2009 H1 N1 vaccine was available for testing by the Food and Drug Administration (FDA), to determine if it was suitable for public release, during the first week of September.

4. **Release.**Tests for concentrations of viral hemagglutinin in inactivated vaccine, using reagents described below (point 6), were completed by the FDA between September 15 and 18.
5. **Fill & finish vaccine.** Initial lots of H1N1 vaccine were placed in syringes and vials or nasal sprayers and packaged by September 30. Given the urgency associated with the developing pandemic, manufacturers shipped 2009 H1N1 vaccines before sterility testing was completed, recognizing that some lots might need to be recalled; no microbial contamination was detected, and the first doses of vaccine were available for clinical use on October 5.

   The supply of H1N1 inactivated vaccine was limited early in the manufacturing phase of the immunization campaign. Approximately 26.7 million doses of this vaccine were available for distribution at the end of October 2009. Because of relatively poor virus production per egg, fewer doses of inactivated vaccine than expected were produced per egg (03-05 doses/egg as compared to the usual 2.0 to 3.0 doses/egg) which contributed to the less than expected supply. Significantly higher numbers of doses of LAIV vaccine were produced per egg (75-100 doses/egg), but only 20% of the total vaccine produced was LAIV because only one fill-finish production line was available up until late October 2009 when a second line became available.[5]

   By mid-November, about 30 million doses of vaccine were ready for use, and about 60 million doses by the end of month. During December, vaccine surpluses replaced shortages, as the supply reached 90 million doses. Afterwards, supplies continued to increase. By the end of February, an estimated 81 to 91 million doses had been administered, covering about a quarter of the US population.

6. **Prepare potency reagents.** The reference virus was provided to the FDA by the CDC on May 26, at the time it was also shipped to manufacturers. The sheep antisera required for potency testing of inactivated vaccines (measurement of HA antigen in immunodiffusion gels) were available August 12.

1-3. Brief Primer on Influenza

Influenza viruses cause frequent widespread infections—annual ("seasonal") epidemics and occasional, potentially severe, world-wide epidemics ("pandemics").These epidemiological patterns are associated with the genetic plasticity of influenza viruses, producing both gradual and sudden changes in genes encoding viral proteins, including the proteins that enable viral entry into and release from cells and the proteins responsible for eliciting the host's immune response. At least two kinds of genetic changes can occur. First, influenza genes are not copied accurately during virus growth; hence many errors (mutations) occur.These small changes (along with the genetic selection that occurs to fix these mutations in the virus) are called "antigenic drift;' and they can affect any of the viral proteins, including major viral surface proteins such as the HA protein that mediates entry into host cells and serves as the major target for the immune response. While antigenic drift may be subtle biochemically, it can have large consequences for the human host, since the immunity acquired from infection during a previous epidemic will not fully protect the host against infection by the new virus. Second, the genes of influenza viruses are present on eight separate segments that together make up the viral RNA genome (in effect, the virus has 8 chromosomes). When two virus particles infect a single cell, the genes of the two viruses can mingle and be efficiently reassorted into the progeny virus. The natural reservoirs for influenza viruses are mostly aquatic birds but they can transmit their viruses to farm animals, such as pigs and ducks. Novel strains infectious for humans can emerge when reassortment occurs among the genetic segments of two or more viruses that have co-infected the various hosts.These major changes, called "antigenic shifts," escape all previous immune protection, contributing to the development of a pandemic when they occur in a virus that is also transmitted efficiently from person to person.

Annual influenza epidemics, known as seasonal influenza, usually occur in late fall and winter in the United States, and take their greatest toll among the elderly and the very young. Seasonal influenza is caused by virus strains that have undergone antigenic drift and differ minimally from strains that have circulated in previous years. In contrast, pandemics, larger-scale epidemics that often affect people in the prime of life, occur whenever a new influenza strain, generally one exhibiting antigenic shift, appears in a largely naive human population and is then transmitted efficiently from one person to another. An influenza pandemic is defined by the number and global distribution of cases, not by the severity of the illness or the percentage of deaths caused by the novel strain.

Influenza vaccines are used to reduce influenza morbidity and mortality by inducing an immune response against viruses predicted to cause seasonal outbreaks or against new viruses isolated early in a wider outbreak that shows signs of developing into a pandemic. Immunization against seasonal influenza viruses compensates for gaps in pre-existing immunity when viruses undergo antigenic drift and for the absence of strain-specific immunity if antigenic shift has occurred to produce a pandemic strain. Vaccines can also provide primary protection for infants and children who have not yet been infected with any influenza viruses.

Both **inactivated and live attenuated** influenza vaccines are approved in the United States. These vaccines are manufactured annually by growth of appropriate strains of virus in embryonated chicken eggs. (In this country, no cell culture-based vaccines or vaccines supplemented with adjuvant are approved for use.) The vaccine strains are developed after surveillance for viruses causing respiratory illness, conducted by the CDC and the WHO network of 120 National Influenza Centers located in more than 90 countries. Early each year, or late in the previous year, the CDC selects component strains for the coming autumn's influenza vaccines to protect against seasonal influenza. Late selection of strains is sometimes necessary and can delay vaccine production, but the period available for manufacturing each annual season's influenza vaccine is usually at least six months.

In contrast, a pandemic strain of influenza virus can emerge at any time, as illustrated by the novel 2009 variant of H1N1. Such strains can cause illnesses outside the usual period of seasonal influenza, provide limited time for vaccine production between the first and second wave of infections, and effectively replace the predicted seasonal strains of virus. All of these phenomena were observed in the 2009 pandemic.

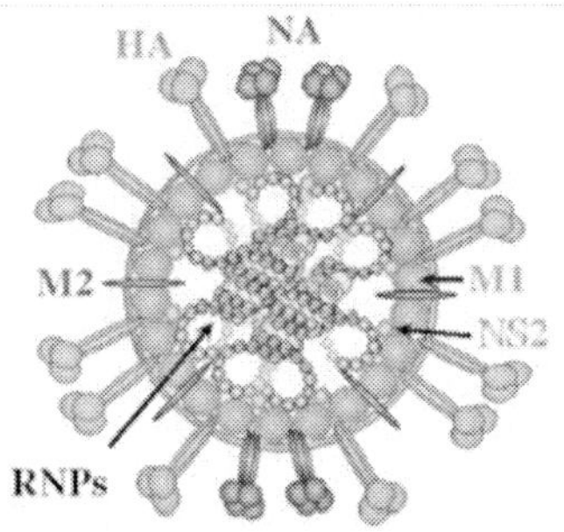

Above is a cartoon depicting a single influenza virus particle, with its eight RNA segments inside as ribonucleoprotein (RNP) surrounded by the major structural proteins of the virus, including the surface proteins neuraminidase (NA) and hemagglutinin (HA) that are used to classify virus strains (e.g. H1N1).

Source: College of St. Benedict/St. John's University.

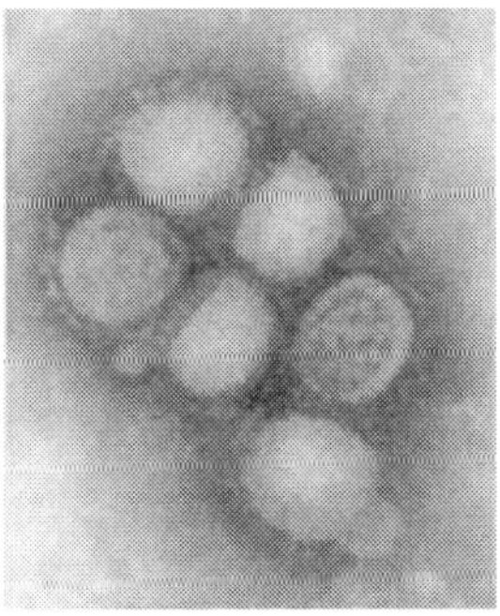

This is a picture of a cluster of six H1N1 influenza virus particles taken with an electron microscope, showing the cores and the spikes of virus surface proteins.

Source: Centers for Disease Control and Prevention.

II. The Influenza Vaccine Problem

Section Summary

Current influenza vaccines are prepared from materials grown in chicken eggs, a cumbersome method that appears out-moded in a world dominated by growth of vaccine viruses in cell culture or by new vaccines designed with recombinant DNA methods. However, proposals to radically change manufacturing processes proven historically to be capable of producing vast quantities of influenza vaccine raise scientific, economic, and regulatory issues that the Federal Government needs to address.

This chapter includes the Working Group's survey of this complex landscape. The chapter first reviews the strategy for dissecting the steps in vaccine preparation in order to determine the sources of difficulty in 2009 and the prospects for improvement in future pandemics. As the reference point for its analysis, the Working Group used the timeline developed by the World Health Organization (WHO) for egg-based production of inactivated influenza vaccine in a pandemic.The chapter then discusses the kinds of choices to be considered and the economic and regulatory barriers to change, and presents the plan for discussing the recommended options.

In particular, the Working Group concluded that because of the commodity nature of influenza vaccine, with its low profit margin, there is little economic incentive for vaccine manufacturers to make major investments in order to change the type of vaccine they manufacture or alter the egg-based process they use to make it. However, there are a number of improvements that the Federal Government and manufacturers can make within the next few years, with little research and development, at relatively low cost, and with no economic impact on manufacturers. These steps include instituting better surveillance to detect new influenza strains earlier, creating stocks of "seed viruses" needed to manufacture vaccines, developing methods to better measure vaccine potency and monitor sterility, and building additional capacity to place vaccine in delivery units.

Improving the prospects for making vaccines against pandemic strains of influenza viruses in a timely fashion requires more than making adjustments to manufacturing procedures. Several steps are involved in the development of a pandemic vaccine, and these depend on public health practices, virology, and the host immune response, as well as manufacturing and packaging of the vaccines. Current influenza vaccines are prepared from materials grown in chicken eggs, a cumbersome method that appears outmoded in a world dominated by production of many viral vaccines in cell culture or by new vaccines designed with recombinant DNA methods. However, proposals to make major changes in large-scale influenza vaccine production technologies in order to protect the nation against an unpredictable risk of pandemic raise economic and regulatory issues that need to be discussed in the context of what is essentially a commodity business dependent on the annual production of smaller amounts of vaccine against seasonal influenza. And because financial incentives for making such changes may seem weak, the government needs to contemplate unusual actions to stimulate, coordinate, and even lead any recommended actions.

This chapter includes PCAST's survey of this complex landscape. The chapter first reviews the strategy for dissecting the steps in vaccine preparation in order to determine the sources of difficulty in 2009 and the prospects for improvement in future pandemics. The chapter then discusses the kinds of choices to be considered and the economic and regulatory barriers to change, and presents a plan for reviewing the recommended options.

Framework for Analysis: Timelines for Vaccine Production

To develop a rigorous analysis of the central question posed by PCAST (see Chapter 1), it has been necessary to identify the components of the vaccine production process and to align possible improvements in those components with the timeline for production. In this way, PCAST has made predictions about the effects of each recommended change on the time to delivery of first doses of vaccine and on the time to delivery of sufficient vaccine to protect 80% of the United States population in a pandemic.

The timeline developed by the WHO for egg-based production of inactivated influenza vaccine in a pandemic serves as a starting point for this analysis (Figure 2-1). This is the major form of influenza vaccine used to protect the United States population against either seasonal or pandemic influenza. The timeline shows the estimated durations of six sets of actions that need to be taken after the isolation and identification of a new strain of influenza virus. Five of these steps are sequential and hence directly determine the time to first dose (about 20 weeks): verification and distribution of the vaccine strain by the CDC; development by manufacturers of an optimized seed strain that encodes the newly identified HA protein and grows well in embryonated eggs; production, inactivation, and quality control of vaccine materials, followed by pooling; permission from the FDA to package and release vaccine for distribution; and filling single-dose syringes or multi-dose vials by the manufacturers. The sixth task, FDA's preparation of reagents for potency testing, usually occurs concordantly with other actions, but if excessively prolonged can also affect the time to delivery of vaccine.

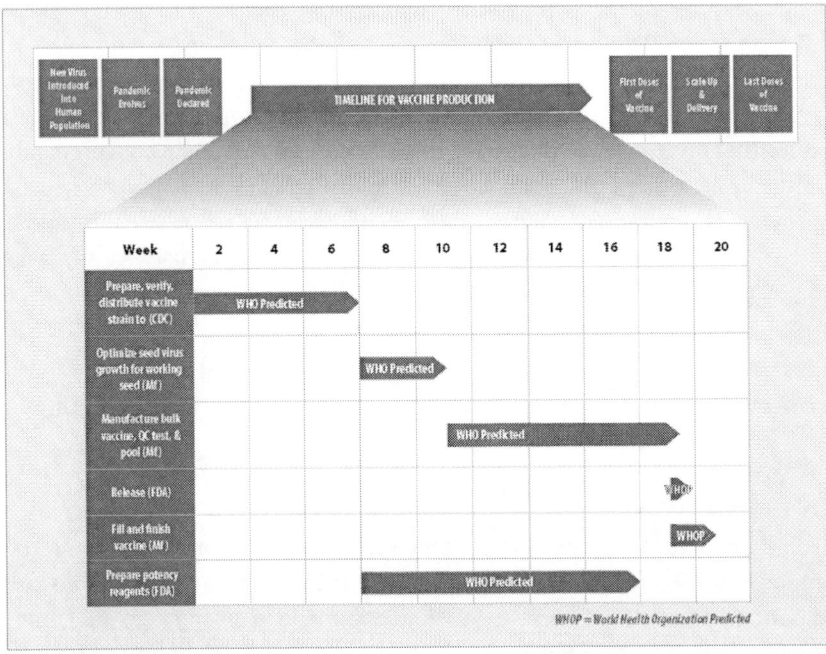

The timeline for an effective vaccine response to a pandemic begins when a new strain of influenza virus causes human disease and serial transmission in the community has been documented. Upon declaration of an epidemic and a decision to produce vaccine to combat it, a series of steps illustrated in the central portion of the figure must be executed. the expected times for performance of each step, as estimated by the WHO for production of egg-based inactivated vaccine, are illustrated by the lengths of each horizontal bar, with the two-color format connoting variation in predicted time. At the tail end of the vaccine production process, manufacturing capacity will determine how much time is required to provide and distribute enough doses to vaccinate 80% of the population. All of the steps shown here, from surveillance to delivery of final doses, are critical for interrupting the spread of the pandemic virus.

Figure 2-1. Timeline for Production of Inactivated Pandemic Influenza Vaccine

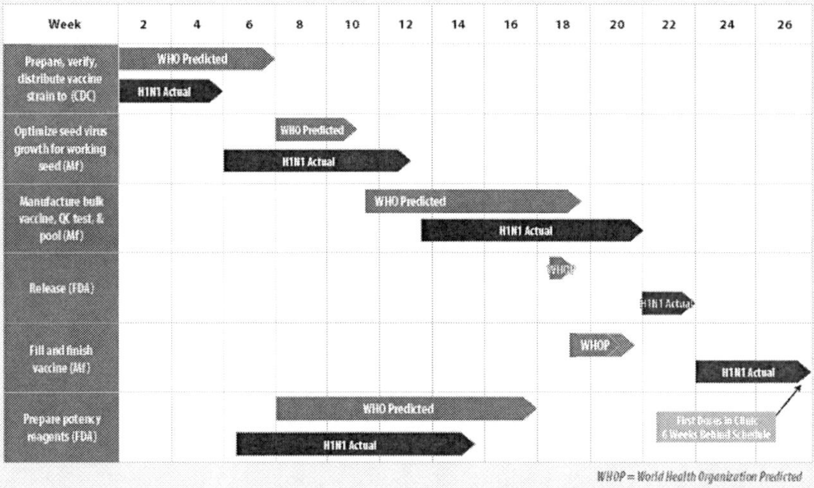

NOTE: This production time line shows time to first doses of inactivated influenza vaccine; time to release of first doses of LAIV was 21 weeks.

This figure compares the actual times and WHO predicted times to complete key steps in the production of 2009 H1N1 egg-based inactivated vaccine. As shown in the top segment, the vaccine seed strain was prepared and distributed to the manufacturers in less time than predicted, but the time needed to optimize this seed strain and prepare a working seed suitable for manufacturing was significantly longer, as seen in the second segment from the top. The preparation of potency reagents necessary for inactivated vaccines was accomplished in a shorter interval than predicted and did not delay release. Initial lots of LAIV were prepared in a shorter time than inactivated influenza vaccine.

Figure 2-2. 2009 H1N1 Vaccine Production Timeline

In addition to the inactivated vaccine, an LAIV vaccine is also approved in the United States, although its use has been more limited. While the initial steps involved in production of this vaccine are similar to those of the inactivated vaccine, production is substantially more efficient for several reasons: potency tests can be eliminated in favor of a simple, rapid determination of the amount of infectious virus in a traditional plaque assay in cultured cells; existing backbones of cold-adapted viruses shorten the preparation of seed strains for attenuated vaccine; and less virus is required per dose of vaccine, reducing production time. Hence, the time to first doses can be shortened slightly, as indicated in the legend to Figure 2-2, whereas time to last dose can be reduced substantially. The time for subsequent production of the doses required to provide full population coverage can vary substantially depending on several key factors, each of which is considered in this chapter: the growth efficiency of the seed strain of virus for vaccine production; the availability of means of production (e.g. embryonated chicken eggs); and the capacity to place the vaccine into the delivery package (e.g. syringes, vials, nasal sprayers).

PCAST used the WHO timeline to help explain the slower-than-desired delivery of vaccine in the 2009 pandemic (Figure 2-2). The major delay in the delivery of first doses was caused by the relatively long time required for the manufacturers to optimize the seed strain supplied by the CDC for growth in eggs. Because production of virus for killed vaccine in eggs inoculated with the working strain was poor, fewer doses of vaccine than usual were produced per egg, markedly increasing the time to produce vaccine in large amounts.

PCAST then examined the possible effects on the timeline of various proposed changes in methodologies. Some changes—in preparation of seed stocks, for example—could improve steps in the timeline by reducing the average length of the step or its variability, even without altering the strategy for vaccine production. Other changes, such as in the means of vaccine production through the use of recombinant DNA technology, could eliminate steps in the timeline.Through this type of analysis, PCAST developed estimates for how much the times for the initial delivery of vaccine and for provision of the full complement of doses might be shortened by the use of improved technologies.These proposed changes and their effects on the delivery of first and last doses of vaccine are described in detail in Chapters 3, 4, and 5.

Weighing Options

Decisions about whether to pursue those improvements and whether to complete them over a certain period of time cannot be made in a vacuum. These decisions need to take into consideration the likelihood of a new pandemic; the potential impacts of pandemics of variable severity in the number of lives, and years of life, that might be saved; the costs to industry and to the Federal Government of making the improvements; and the feasibility of success in achieving recommended goals.

In particular, the investment required by the Federal Government to ensure each potential action described in this chapter must be estimated, and making such an estimate requires understanding the economics of the vaccine market.

Manufacturers may lack sufficient economic motivation to invest in actions that may be useful only in the case of a pandemic, and even then they may not realize a substantial economic return on that investment. For this reason, the Federal Government may need to provide substantial economic incentives to enhance preparedness for an influenza pandemic. To recommend such incentives, the potential benefits of each action must be balanced against the likely cost to the Federal Government and evaluated with respect to the likelihood and probable pace of progress in developing the next generation of vaccine production technologies. In addition, a plan for coordination and oversight of such efforts would be needed to ensure that the program is executed in a timely and responsible manner.

The benefits that may result from reducing the number of weeks to initial vaccination cannot be predicted accurately. However, as an illustration, one study indicates that in the relatively mild 2009 H1 N1 pandemic, an additional 2,200 lives could have been saved in the United States if vaccinations had started one month earlier.[6] It is important, in making such calculations, to remember that in comparison with seasonal flu the 2009-H1 N1 pandemic had a much greater impact on younger individuals—more than 85% of the deaths during the 2009 H1 N1 pandemic were in people younger than 60, with an overall mean age of 37.4 years, as compared to an overall mean age of 75.7 years for victims of seasonal influenza. The benefits of delivering vaccine early, of course, also include reducing the overall burden of morbidity and disruption caused by a pandemic and potentially reducing the likelihood of recurrent waves of infection.[7] Finally, Federal funds used to support the development of new influenza vaccine manufacturing platforms and facilities (and thus enhance our capacity to respond to pandemics) could potentially enhance our ability to develop medical countermeasures against other novel pathogens.

It is difficult, if not impossible, to undertake this analysis in a fully rigorous and quantitative manner. Nonetheless, a framework for decision-making can help clarify the issues. For example, egg-based influenza vaccines are not an adequate long-term solution for responding to a pandemic, mainly because, as occurred in 2009, the complete process may fail to provide adequate vaccine in time to block the second wave of disease. Nonetheless, egg-based production of a combination of killed vaccine and LAIV vaccine is currently the only FDA-approved technology with sufficient capacity to supply enough doses for the entire United States population; this will probably remain the case for at least three years and possibly more. For this reason, it is easy to justify modest investments, such as developing a set of viral backbones for making seed stocks rapidly or increasing the use of LAIVs vaccines, that could significantly shorten the time to respond to a pandemic with egg-based vaccines.

Shifts to new technologies for vaccine production, including cell culture-based vaccines or vaccines derived from recombinant DNA methods, present greater complexities in decision-making. While a switch to cell culture for virus growth will not materially accelerate the time to first dose, it can significantly accelerate the time to last dose because cell-based production of virus is more readily scaled up than egg-based production. The vaccines produced in cell culture are essentially identical to currently approved egg-grown vaccines, both inactivated or LAIV. However, cell culture-based influenza vaccines have not been approved by the FDA, and turning to cell culture systems will likely require construction of additional facilities to permit adequate levels of production even with a major production shift from inactivated vaccines to the more efficiently produced LAIV vaccines, as discussed in Chapter 4.

Recombinant DNA technology would significantly shorten both the time to first dose and the time to last dose because it eliminates the need for seed strains of virus and speeds up production of viral antigen. However, no recombinant influenza vaccine has been FDA approved, technological risks remain unresolved, and safety and efficacy of recombinant vaccines must be demonstrated.These uncertainties create a dilemma for decision-makers that is discussed more fully in Chapter 5.

Addition of immune stimulants (adjuvants) to certain vaccines can make vaccines more effective, allowing smaller amounts of viral material to be used per dose of vaccine (thereby, in effect, accelerating production). However, these gains need to be balanced against uncertainties about safety and acceptance of adjuvanted vaccines and the possibility of developing better adjuvants in the near future, as described in Chapter 6. A universal influenza vaccine that could provide lifelong protection against a wide range of influenza strains would clearly be the optimal solution, but current knowledge does not allow a prediction of whether such a vaccine will ever be possible. With the goal of developing a universal vaccine in mind, substantial investments in basic research as part of a portfolio seem sensible, as discussed in Chapter 7, but large investments in a universal vaccine strategy as part of a preparedness plan is difficult to justify.

A key consideration in this analysis is the over-arching uncertainty as to when the next serious influenza pandemic may occur. During the past 100 years, there were four influenza pandemics (in 1918, 1957, 1968, and 2009), and the death tolls in the US were estimated to have been, respectively, 5000,

1000, 170, and 50 deaths per million inhabitants. Given this frequency, it is possible that no serious pandemic will occur during the next decade or two, providing appreciable time to develop new vaccine strategies for pandemics while depending on current egg-based vaccines for protection against seasonal influenza. However, this may be a highly misleading estimate of pandemic frequencies and severities. Increased travel and migration and the growing intensity of farming birds and swine (critical reservoirs for influenza), particularly in the developing world, may enhance the rate of viral spread and evolution, thereby promoting pandemics, and a pandemic of avian influenza might be more virulent or transmissible between humans than it has been in most previous outbreaks. Although it is impossible to predict with any certainty, the Federal Government might assume, solely for planning purposes, at least a 3 percent per annum probability of an influenza pandemic; a pandemic that caused 1000 deaths per million would translate to 300,000 deaths in the United States. Given these assumed probabilities and potential consequences, it would seem reasonable for the Federal Government to invest at least $1 billion per year to prevent such an outcome.

Economics of Vaccine Manufacture

Influenza vaccine manufacturing is a commodity business, with little differentiation among products and consequently relatively low profit margins. The United States population is served by five major influenza vaccine manufacturers: Sanofi-Pasteur, Novartis, GlaxoSmithKline, MedImmune, and CSL. Of these, only MedImmune makes LAIV vaccine; the others produce killed vaccines. In a typical year, only about one-third of the United States population receives seasonal influenza vaccine, corresponding to a total annual US market size of between 80-100 million doses. The difficulties of predicting how many people will take the vaccine each year and of timing the supply to match peak demand can result in the production of millions of excess doses of vaccines each year. Manufacturers absorb the cost of those unused vaccines through rebates to purchasers.

Manufacturers typically receive a wholesale price of about $5-10 per dose for seasonal influenza vaccine; doses that reach the market earlier in the season command a slightly higher price, which declines over the season.The precise profit margin is proprietary information, but knowledgeable observers estimate that it is about 20 percent (reflecting the costs of the considerable manual labor involved in egg-based production, the cost of filling syringes, and the annual rebates). A manufacturer with 50 percent market share might thus net about $30 million in annual profit.

By contrast, pharmaceutical companies typically have profit margins of 50-95 percent, with the highest margins for novel, proprietary drugs. Such large profit margins for novel drugs are the norm because of lower competition, and companies justify them as a means to recover the costs involved in developing and testing drugs and securing regulatory approval. The high return-on-investment for these products affects manufacturers' willingness to invest capital in a commodity business such as influenza vaccine; such investments are often evaluated against the "opportunity costs" of alternative investments with higher returns.

Nevertheless, it is in the national interest to improve preparedness for an influenza pandemic, even though substantial investment in innovations and substantial economic risks may be required to create a new vaccine that can reduce the timeline for production. Manufacturers have a limited economic incentive to invest in such innovations for seasonal influenza vaccines, because there is much less time pressure in the preparation for seasonal influenza than for a pandemic.

To induce existing manufacturers to shift to vaccine production methods that would allow a rapid response in the event of future sporadic pandemics, the Federal Government may need to cover a significant fraction of the cost of such innovations and take an active role in convening and coordinating work with the multiple pharmaceutical and biotechnology companies engaged in the development and production of influenza vaccines. For example, building a new cell culture-based vaccine manufacturing facility may cost more than $1 billion. With annual profits of only $30 million, it would take over 30 years to recover the investment in nominal dollars (leaving aside the need for a return on investment). Novartis recently constructed such a facility in Holly Springs, North Carolina.To partially offset the cost, the Department of Health and Human Services provided $497 million in Federal funding.

While manufacturers have limited incentives to invest solely to reduce timelines, there may be synergies that could provide some incentives for investment. For example, some innovations that reduce timelines may also result in improved, more desirable, and hence more widely used products (such as those that provide better protection of the elderly, who are at particular risk during epidemics of seasonal influenza). Some innovations may also decrease manufacturing costs (leading to a higher profit margin for the manufacturers that adopt them).

Finally, serious regulatory issues can impede innovation. Uncertain pathways to secure FDA approval for cell culture-based vaccines, recombinant vaccines, and vaccines containing adjuvants inhibit investment, because manufacturers may not know whether or when they could expect to bring such vaccines to market. Provision of clear regulatory guidance by the FDA would be one of the most important—and least expensive—steps to lower barriers to innovation in influenza vaccine production.

Components of a National Response: An Overview

Several types of improvements can be envisioned in the methods that contribute to the production of pandemic (and seasonal) influenza vaccines. Some of these, such as better ways to detect new strains, make seed stocks, control vaccine potency, monitor sterility, and place vaccine in delivery devices, could be instituted in the near future. When taken in concert, these improvements could advance the starting point for vaccine production by several weeks and reduce the WHO time course to delivery of first doses (see Chapter 3). Moreover, such improved methods may be applied to the manufacturing of influenza vaccines by different means (in eggs, in cell culture, or by recombinant technologies) and sometimes to other vaccines and medical problems. In this sense, they may constitute"platform technologies"and are so noted when presented in Chapter 3.

Other changes represent more fundamental alterations in the mode of production of influenza vaccines. Transformation of production of a vaccine strain of virus from an egg-based to a cell culture based industry would not, by itself, have a major effect on the time to delivery of first doses, but could dramatically reduce the time to delivery of last doses by half or more, because of the rapid scale-up of growth. A change from killed-virus vaccine to LAIV vaccine would also shorten the time to last doses by reducing the amount of virus required for each dose of vaccine by up to one hundred fold. However, only one manufacturer is licensed to make LAIV vaccine, and the methodology is proprietary to that company. A more radical change in design of influenza vaccines to a method based on recombinant DNA technology could have even greater effects, since at least one time-consuming step, the preparation of seed stocks of virus, would be eliminated and the scale-up in production of vaccine materials (in this case, proteins encoded by viral nucleic acids) could together shorten the time to delivery of first doses to 13 weeks.

The attractions and difficulties of making these major changes are discussed in Chapter 5.

Two other scientific and technological issues could have important effects on the production and use of influenza vaccines. Adjuvants could significantly reduce the amount of antigenic material required in any type of influenza vaccine and thereby shorten the time required to provide all of the necessary doses. As considered in Chapter 6, there are substantial obstacles—scientific, regulatory, and commercial—to adoption of adjuvanted vaccines, but approval of such vaccines in other countries, improved adjuvants, and better understanding of the mechanisms by which they augment the immune response all argue for greater use of adjuvants in influenza vaccines in the future. In addition, it remains plausible to envision influenza vaccines that induce a more durable and more broadly cross-reactive immune response, thereby eliminating the need for yearly vaccinations against seasonal influenza and offering better protection against new pandemic strains of virus. Strategies for developing such vaccines and the kinds of fundamental research required to encourage development are outlined in Chapter 7.

Finally, wide-ranging efforts to hasten and improve the production of influenza vaccines will require unaccustomed levels of coordination among government agencies, academic scientists, and the industrial sector, as well as investments of public funds as part of a package of incentives. Such planning and spending can only be achieved by assigning implementation and oversight to responsible components of the Federal Government or to a government-chartered entity. Recommendations for doing this are presented in Chapter 8.

The effects of PCAST's recommendations on the delivery of pandemic influenza vaccines are summarized in Table 2-1 on the following page.

Table 2-1. Effects of Recomended Actions on Delivery of Pandemic Influenza Vaccines

Recommended Change	Estimated Time Required to Make the Change	Effects on Time to First Dose	Effects on Bulk Production Until Demand Satisfied	Alternative Uses in Medical Countermea sures
Increased Surveillance	1-3 years	Moves the starting line forward by weeks or more	None	Yes

Table 2-1. (Continued)

Recommended Change	Estimated Time Required to Make the Change	Effects on Time to First Dose	Effects on Bulk Production Until Demand Satisfied	Alternative Uses in Medical Countermeasures
Faster Production of Optimal Vaccine Seed	1-2 years	Up to several weeks	Up to several weeks (if more efficient virus growth)	No
Modernized Sterility Tests	1-2 years	Approximately 1 week	None	Yes
Improved Generation of Potency Reagents	1-2 years	Avoids possible delay of up to several weeks	None	Possibly
Expanded and Streamlined Fill and Finish Procedures	1-3 years	Slight	Up to weeks	Yes
Shift to Cell Culture to make Killed Vaccine	1-3 years	A few weeks	Up to several weeks	Possibly
Shift to Cell Culture for Live Attenuated Vaccine	2-6 years	A few weeks	Up to several weeks	Possibly
Recombinant–based Vaccine	2-10 years	Several weeks	Up to several weeks	Yes

III. Potential Benefits of Short Term Changes in Methods for Making Influenza Vaccines

Section Summary

A major lesson of the 2009 H1N1 influenza pandemic is that the supply of vaccine sufficient to protect the United States population is vulnerable to delays at the beginning of the process, when the vaccine virus must be optimized for manufacturing, and at the end of the process, during the final fill-finish packaging of the vaccine.The decision to begin influenza vaccine production depends on surveillance for early detection of a new influenza strain. Global surveillance for emerging influenza viruses requires no new technology, but does need better coordination among the WHO, CDC, and local hospitals and diagnostic laboratories and wider dissemination of modern viral detection technologies. An investment in developing new viral backbones optimized for growth in chicken eggs or mammalian cell culture would lessen the chances that seed viruses will grow poorly when put into production and likely increase vaccine yields, reducing the time needed to produce enough vaccine to immunize all of the Nation's residents. Potency testing of inactivated influenza vaccine relies on an outmoded technology prone to delays, but with a focused research effort it should be possible to adapt contemporary methods for use during the vaccine manufacturing process. Sterility testing can also be done more rapidly with recently developed technologies. No new technologies are needed to substantially reduce the fill-finish bottleneck, but industry and the Federal government must develop a plan and identify the necessary financial resources to ensure adequate capacity to produce sufficient quantities of pre-filled syringes, vials, and/or nasal sprayers to meet the national need.

As described in Section 2, the several steps involved in the development and production of pandemic influenza vaccines are predicted to require an average of about 20 weeks after isolation of the pandemic strain until the first doses of vaccine are available from manufacturers. Chapter 2 also noted that the supply of vaccine sufficient to protect the entire population is susceptible to delays in virus growth, in the final fill-finish packaging of the vaccine, and other vulnerabilities. PCAST has considered ways to improve each of these steps and has found that most can be improved in the relatively near future, possibly within the next three years if funds are available and regulatory issues are addressed.This chapter outlines steps that can be taken in the short term, describes how some of the improvements can help establish platform technologies applicable to a variety of situations involving biological threats, and envisions the impacts of the proposed improvements on the time to delivery of first and last doses of pandemic vaccine. In the following chapters, proposals for transfer of vaccine production to cell culture and the longer term potential of recombinant technology for making influenza vaccines are discussed.

Surveillance

The initial trigger for assessing whether a pandemic vaccine will be needed is the identification of a novel influenza virus exhibiting antigenic shift and circulating in the human population. The transmissibility of the novel virus is a key criterion for declaration of a global pandemic, which is the responsibility of WHO. This declaration happens, as in the 2009 influenza pandemic, when an unusual cluster of cases of influenza-like illnesses is noted by public health workers and patient samples are then sent to a diagnostic laboratory capable of identifying subtypes of influenza virus. Even if a novel virus proves not to be readily transmissible, the first steps towards developing seed strains for possible use as a vaccine are not costly and can be undertaken well before the decision about declaring a pandemic is made.

Surveillance precedes the starting point for the timelines shown in Figure 2-1, and therefore does not directly affect assessments of the time required for vaccine production that begins with the declaration of a pandemic and ends with delivery of vaccine. However, earlier detection of an influenza virus with pandemic potential has obvious benefits. The likelihood that surveillance will detect new pathogens more effectively can be increased by widening the use of surveillance methods geographically, by lowering the criteria for collecting and submitting samples to a reference laboratory, and, when appropriate, by testing animal as well as human hosts. In this way surveillance can lengthen the time available for making enough vaccine to protect the population. In 2009, identification of the new H1N1 and tracking its transmissibility in the human population even two months earlier would have allowed the first doses of vaccine to be delivered before the next wave of the pandemic began in late August and might have interrupted this second wave, which peaked in the fall before vaccine was widely available.

Since better surveillance accelerates the decision to make a pandemic vaccine, it is a fundamental component of pandemic preparedness. A cluster of unexplained illnesses or deaths is usually the first marker of an incipient pandemic. Although the expectation has been that influenza strains with pandemic potential will emerge in Asia, clusters of influenza-like illness subsequently attributed to the novel 2009-H1 N1 virus were first identified in Mexico and the United States, supporting the importance of comprehensive global surveillance. Much can be done to recognize and spread the news about such clusters, given contemporary global communications tools. One approach would be to further develop an integrated Web-based system for electronic reporting of unexpected numbers of patients with respiratory illnesses outside the usual influenza season or with unusual disease profiles, e.g., greater severity, unexpected complications, or higher attack rates among young adults rather than the elderly during the usual influenza season.

Recognition of illness clusters is not useful without efficient collection and shipping of patient materials to reference laboratories for diagnostic testing. The WHO influenza surveillance network has made influenza diagnostic reagents and polymerase chain reaction (PCR) equipment to detect influenza viruses more widely available in recent years. This infrastructure helped to demonstrate quickly the global reach of the 2009 H1N1 pandemic. Enhancing the capacity of these centers to rapidly identify non-subtypable influenza viruses in patients and report those finding to WHO reference laboratories or to the CDC could reduce substantially the timeline for recognizing an emerging pandemic. The United States Agency for International Development (USAID), the Department of Defense (DoD), and national public health programs in any country at risk could also contribute in useful ways to the development of more effective surveillance networks.

Reinforcing current disease detection and laboratory diagnostic networks is feasible in the short term, but novel technologies that are simple, sensitive, precise, rapid, and designed for use in resource-poor settings are needed for global distribution. The goal of such innovation should be a sustainable, multi-use respiratory disease surveillance platform, deployable worldwide, for rapid detection by reverse transcription PCR (RT-PCR) sequencing or proteomics methods to detect major changes in existing human influenza strains as well as influenza H2, H4, H6, H7, H9, and H10 Type A influenza viruses that constitute pandemic threats. Such technologies have broad applications for identifying other emerging infections as well and hence qualify as multi-use platforms for emergency preparedness. Where appropriate, these platforms should leverage standardized diagnostic platforms for infectious agents now being developed, such as the Next Generation Diagnostic System that is being funded in the FY 2011 budget of the DOD.

New influenza viruses that threaten the human population emerge from animal reservoirs, either directly or more often by transfer of parts of the viral genome into co-existing viruses already adapted to infect people. Surveillance of wild birds, domestic poultry, and pigs with multi-use platform technology for respiratory viruses by the United States Department of Agriculture (USDA), other US agencies, and agriculture and wild life programs of other nations could lead to early recognition of influenza strains with pandemic potential. Meanwhile, progress could be made using existing detection methods if disincentives for agricultural surveillance and global collaboration were addressed. These disincentives include concerns about the real threat of commercial impact, including disruption of businesses and tourism, and about national jurisdiction and control over the information and materials resulting from surveillance.

RECOMMENDATION 3-1. SURVEILLANCE FOR AND IDENTIFICATION OF NOVEL VIRUSES

The CDC should develop improved strategies for global influenza surveillance, taking advantage of the existing CDC/WHO collaboration and considering additional partnerships with USAID, DoD, USDA, other United States agencies, and foreign public health systems.These strategies should be implemented within two years and should include:

- Pursuing improvements that enhance global networks for electronic reporting of clusters of cases of respiratory illness that are atypical of seasonal influenza; this type of surveillance is symptom-based and does not require immediate access to a diagnostic laboratory.
- Developing and assessing innovative approaches that exploit contemporary communications tools, including cell phones and the Internet, or that expedite reporting of novel cases and clusters of respiratory illness.
- Improving rapid collection and transfer of patient specimens to WHO influenza reference laboratories.
- Supporting better global access to PCR-based detection of novel respiratory pathogens.
- Increasing surveillance of certain animals known to be natural hosts for influenza viruses, especially pigs and some domestic fowl.

In addition, the National Institute of Allergy and Infectious Diseases (NIAID), Biomedical Advanced Research and Development Authority (BARDA), and CDC should support innovation grants and contracts to academic and private sector teams for new multi-use technologies to detect novel respiratory viruses with pandemic potential and consider coordination with similar programs supported by the DOD.The focus should be on platform technologies with the capacity to detect other infectious agents as well as influenza viruses.

Development of Influenza Vaccine Seed Strains

At present, influenza vaccines approved in the United States must be manufactured in eggs, yet influenza viruses that infect humans often grow poorly in eggs.Therefore, developing a vaccine seed virus entails creating a hybrid virus containing viral genes coding for the new HA and neuraminidase (N) proteins in a backbone of other influenza genes that help the virus to infect eggs. Creating these vaccine seed strains (also known as reassortants) is achieved by mixing the new influenza strain with a virus adapted to infect eggs and monitoring virus progeny for gene swapping after infection of eggs with both viruses. The seed strain for LAIV differs from that required to make the killed virus vaccine; LAIV must be made by swapping the new HA and N genes into an existing genetically defined influenza backbone that is adapted to grow at the lower temperature of the nasal passages where the vaccine is delivered. It is also impaired, or attenuated, for growth at the higher body temperature of the lung. In either case, the basic problem for preparing vaccine seed strains for manufacturing is that effects on growth are unpredictable when HA and N genes from one influenza virus are recombined with the other six genes of another strain because functions of these genes are influenced by the context provided by other viral genes. The difficulties of creating a high titer seed strain, especially one that will grow efficiently when scaled up for manufacturing, can cause significant delays in the time line for first delivery of pandemic influenza vaccines, as was the case with the 2009 H1N1 vaccine.

Reassortent techniques are readily applicable to deriving influenza seed strains because of the ease with which influenza viruses exchange genes (see Box 1-3). However, contemporary molecular genetic methods can be used to optimize this process and can be applied to create viral recombinants that grow more efficiently in embryonated eggs or in cultured cells used to produce influenza vaccines in Europe (see Chapter 4). Even though the viral backbone remains the same for each LAIV product, reverse genetic methods are also applicable in this context because the novel HA gene can be manipulated to minimize interference with vaccine virus growth.

Given the many years of experience with developing vaccine seed strains that grow well and the availability of these seed viruses, along with contemporary rapid sequencing tools, research can be undertaken to better understand the interactions of influenza genes and should make the behavior of influenza reassortants more predictable with respect to likely growth in eggs. It should be feasible, for example, to develop libraries of backbone viruses that can be used to make reassortants with new HA and N genes for the manufacture of inactivated vaccines, and the reassortants can then be screened rapidly to identify those with the best growth characteristics. If the transition to cell culture production moves forward in the United States, similar molecular approaches can be used to derive a panel of influenza backbones with good growth potential in cultured cells.

Genetic methods can also be used to test HA and N genes for minor mutations (outside the major antigenic regions of HA) that are associated with better yields, despite their transfer into a non-native influenza genome. Making LAIV requires that the backbone remain unmodified so that the vaccine virus retains the cold-adapted, temperature-sensitive-characteristics needed for optimum safety and effectiveness.Therefore, there is substantial experience with the consequences on viral growth of introducing novel HA and N genes into this backbone. Such reassortants are a resource for understanding how to optimize growth by making minor modifications of the HA gene when it is necessary to swap in new HA and N genes to make a pandemic vaccine.

The opportunity also exists to make libraries of influenza seed strains with good growth characteristics that have HA and N genes from influenza viruses considered to have pandemic potential and store these reassortants for immediate use in manufacturing if the need arises.

RECOMMENDATION 3-2. DEVELOP OPTIMIZED SEED VIRUSES

NIAID and BARDA should ensure the development and dissemination of a panel of viral backbones to create seed viruses optimized for rapid growth. Such backbones can accelerate production of inactivated vaccines either in eggs or in mammalian cell culture. Studies of HA and N genes in the context of these backbones and in the LAIV backbone should also be pursued to maximize growth.This should be accomplished through focused contracts, with the aim of producing such viral backbones within 2-3 years.

Potency Testing of Influenza Vaccines during Production and Release

A critical step in manufacture of many vaccines, including inactivated influenza vaccines, is testing vaccine material to determine the concentration of correctly folded antigen (immuno-reactive protein). This is referred to as "potency" testing, although it actually measures the amount of physical material that reacts with antibodies, rather than its true ability to induce an effective immune response when the standard 15 microgram dose of HA antigen in the inactivated vaccine is ad ministered.These measurements are necessary for manufacturers to monitor production of the vaccine strain during virus growth in eggs (or cell culture) and for the FDA to authorize the release of pooled lots of vaccines. Although not a direct test of immunogenicity, vaccines that fail the criteria for release based on potency testing are expected to be poorly immunogenic in many vaccine recipients. The potency of LAIV is determined by a rapid, standard plaque assay in cultured cells; this test measures the concentration of infectious virus—also not a direct test of immunogenicity—but it does not require the generation of immunological reagents that sometimes impedes the production and release of inactivated vaccines.

The method currently used to detect HA in inactivated vaccines requires sheep antisera containing antibodies that bind to the novel HA antigen in its native state. To make this key reagent, sheep are immunized with the new HA antigen to produce large quantities of antisera against HA. Under current practice, the CDC provides the reference (pre-seed) influenza virus to the FDA, which is then responsible for making purified HA to immunize sheep and for overseeing production of the HA antiserum. The amount of HA in a sample of inactivated vaccine is then determined using a radial immunodiffusion assay, a method first described in 1957.The sheep antiserum is suspended in agar and a test specimen from the bulk vaccine is placed in a well cut in the agar; the antigen diffuses from the well and binds to HA antibodies in the agar, forming a visible circle around the well. The amount of HA in the vaccine is calculated from the diameter of the circle.

Though this process may sound straightforward, problems with making potency reagents are a well- known source of delays in manufacturing seasonal influenza vaccines, since serious bottlenecks in production and delivery can occur if effective reagents are not available when vaccine materials are ready for testing and packaging.The time needed to make sheep antisera varies from 8-12 weeks (see Figure 2-1), depending on the time that it takes for the animals to mount an immune response to the specific HA. Moreover, the quality of the HA antiserum that an immunized animal will produce is unpredictable. If the HA antibodies are of low affinity, it may be necessary to repeat the process in other animals.

Approaches to develop faster and more predictable methods to generate reagents and measure HA content could reduce the risk of delaying vaccine release; some of these would be applicable not only to inactivated vaccines against multiple types of influenza viruses, but also to certain vaccines for other infectious agents. Such strategies might eliminate the need to immunize sheep and thereby hasten the availability of antisera for potency testing. In addition, antigen for immunization might be produced more quickly—for example, by cloning a newly identified HA gene into an expression vector to generate large quantities of recombinant HA in mammalian cells for immunizing animals.The use of antisera raised with recombinant HA would, of course, need to be validated in the radial immunodiffusion assay using previously tested vaccine material. These reagents can also be coupled to more contemporary biochemical or physico-chemical platforms for measurement of HA concentration, such as enzyme immunoassays or immunoprecipitation/ mass spectroscopy assays. Work done by the Centers for Disease Control suggests that isotope dilution mass spectrometry methods could be used to reduce substantially the time to measure the antigen content of influenza vaccines and thus make influenza vaccines available 4-8 weeks earlier. Additional work incorporating antibody capture of antigen prior to mass spectrometry analysis will be published soon. Compared to the current potency assay, the antibody- capture mass spectrometry method provides better selectivity for different influenza antigens, better accuracy and precision, shorter analysis time and better sensitivity that enables direct analysis of the small amounts of antigen in vaccines, including adjuvant-based vaccines for the first time.[8] The time to availability might be reduced even more decisively by preparing panels of HA antibody reagents in advance, using phage libraries or pre-synthesized panels of monoclonal antibodies against HA molecules from influenza viruses identified as potential pandemic strains. These reagents would be ready to screen for reactivity against HA made by the newly identified virus in infected cells or the cloned HA gene and used in antibody-based assays to measure the HA content of vaccine preparations. Validation of these approaches to meet regulatory requirements would be necessary.

Another rationale for developing these methods and reagents is their potential application to the problem of understanding the reasons for HA instability in some influenza vaccines; loss of potency was encountered with some lots of 2009-H1N1 vaccine. Potency testing will also be necessary for use with the second generation influenza vaccines based on recombinant DNA technologies, discussed in Chapter 5.

Recommendation 3-3. Potency Testing

FDA and BARDA should fund applied research to develop rapid methods for making potency assays for testing inactivated influenza vaccines. This should be a high-priority effort carried out through a combination of in-house programs at FDA and contracts to companies, aimed at creating and implementing such methods within a 2-3 year time frame. Possible methods include mass spectroscopy coupled with molecular biological techniques for making affinity reagents. Such methods will need to be carefully validated by comparison with the standard radial immunodiffusion assay.

In addition, FDA should develop a well-defined regulatory process for introducing alternative assays for HA potency for seasonal influenza vaccines, initially alongside existing assays.

SterilityTesting

Each batch of vaccine material must be tested to ensure that it is not contaminated with bacteria or fungi, a recurrent problem in egg-based manufacture and one that can also occur when vaccine is prepared in cell culture. Sterility testing is currently accomplished by incubating vaccine material in conventional growth media and waiting to observe bacterial or fungal growth, a process that typically takes about two weeks. It is possible to ship the vaccine while awaiting the results of sterility testing, although the vaccine cannot be administered until the testing is completed.

New, more rapid sterility testing methods are feasible. These methods include PCR and sequencing or array-based technologies using reagents that will identify a wide range of organisms, and rapid, massively parallel sequencing to detect microbes without prior assumptions about what contaminants may be present. Use of such molecular techniques to test directly for microbial contamination could reduce the time to release a batch of vaccine by at least one week, could be more sensitive, and could be applicable to many kinds of vaccines and biologicals, not just influenza vaccines, and hence constitute a multi-use platform technology.

RECOMMENDATION 3-4. DEVELOP PLATFORM TECHNOLOGY FOR STERILITY TESTING

The FDA and BARDA should support the development of rapid methods to test the sterility of influenza vaccines, through such molecular biological techniques as PCR and shotgun DNA sequencing. This should be carried out through private sector contracts and in collaboration with manufacturers.

The methods should be performed in parallel with existing sterility testing of seasonal influenza vaccines, to demonstrate the sensitivity and validity of the methods.

The FDA should define a regulatory process to guide development and implementation.

Manufacturing Fill-Finish Capacity

All vaccines must be packaged for clinical use. The fill-finish step for inactivated influenza vaccines involves transferring bulk vaccine into individual single-dose syringes as well as the single or multi-dose vials used for inactivated influenza vaccines or to nasal sprayers required for the live attenuated vaccines. This step is a major hurdle on the path to vaccine distribution to providers. It represents a costly and laborious phase of manufacturing that can be expanded only in a linear fashion, and it generally proves to be a major rate-limiting step in the process of delivering vaccine, especially under pandemic conditions. The effects of delays in the fill-finish step are felt mainly as production is scaled-up, with little effect on the time to delivery of first doses. Packaging a greater proportion of vaccine in multi-dose vials could eliminate several weeks from the time needed to deliver all of the needed doses of vaccine, but the savings in time must be balanced against the increased risk of contamination of the vial or inadvertent failure to change needles between doses; moreover, multi-dose vials generally require the inclusion of preservatives.

Greater capacity can also be achieved by the construction and validation of additional facilities with more machines for sterile filling and finishing, but the additional costs for such added facilities will not be readily absorbed by the manufacturers. Use of facilities and filling machines that can process different vaccines at different times of the year would expand fill-finish capacity at a less onerous expense, but guidance from regulators would be required to avoid safety violations and delays in manufacturing. Having agreements to allow rapid transfer of production facilities to pandemic vaccine production could be done in advance, possibly including providing a retainer to companies in order to maintain this capability. Developing pre-approved options for nasal administration in addition to sprayers could reduce the barrier to rapid distribution of live attenuated vaccines. Improving the machinery that performs all of these tasks may also be possible, and government incentives to promote such advances in manufacturing should be considered, especially if they can be designed as multi-use platforms.

Today, fill-finish to meet the Nation's demand for seasonal influenza vaccines is done at four facilities in the United States, as well as three facilities outside of the Nation's borders. Options for sustaining or rapidly mobilizing facility and personnel capacity needed for this critical task need to be studied further.

Recommendation 3-5. Fill-Finish Capacity

The Federal Government, working closely with manufacturers, should undertake a comprehensive study within six months to quantitatively assess current fill-finish capacity and to develop a plan to ensure adequate capacity to produce sufficient quantities of pre-filled syringes, vials and/or nasal sprayers to meet the national need. The study should evaluate the use of existing facilities or the creation of new facilities that could be used in the event of a pandemic, including necessary agreements, preparations and licensure. It should also address maintaining a sufficient stockpile of vaccine containers and delivery devices.

IV. Production of Influenza Vaccines in Cultured Cells

Section Summary

Today, all influenza vaccine used in the United States is made by growing the selected viral vaccine strains in embryonated chicken eggs. Alternative methods for producing influenza vaccines, using mammalian cell culture (or, as discussed in Chapter 5, recombinant DNA technology), are in development, and each has the potential to make vaccine production more reliable and faster.

Expansion of the capacity to produce influenza vaccine in mammalian cell culture would permit more rapid scale-up in the face of a pandemic, thereby shortening the time for production of sufficient quantities of vaccine needed to protect the United States population. However, such expansion faces fiscal and regulatory uncertainties that need to be fully understood and alleviated. An important aspect of such an assessment includes evaluating the barriers to the use of LAIV produced in cell culture, possibly permitting a more efficient use of existing production facilities.

Today, the only approved method for making either inactivated influenza or LAIV vaccines for use in the United States involves the production of the selected viral strains in embryonated chicken eggs. In principle, however, influenza vaccines can be prepared using viruses grown in cultured cells or using proteins made with recombinant DNA methods. A number of these technologies are currently in various stages of development. Shifting the method of production and/or in the composition of the vaccines can markedly affect the time course for delivery of vaccines and the reliability of delivery. These possible changes are considered in detail in this and the following chapters.

Cell Culture-Based Production

The change in approach to vaccine production most likely to have an impact in the short term involves producing vaccine viruses in cell culture-based propagation systems rather than in embryonated chicken eggs. Cell culture-based systems would be used to produce the same kind of vaccines that are currently made, i.e., whole disrupted (inactive) virus as well as genetically attenuated virus (LAIV), and hence will pose less biological uncertainty and fewer regulatory difficulties than recombinant influenza vaccines (see Chapter 5). A transition to cell culture-based production has been under consideration for many years, and several companies are proceeding to develop and commercialize vaccine produced by this method. Cell culture production alone provides some improvements in time to first dose in the event of a pandemic, but does not alleviate the earlier potential bottlenecks such as optimization of an appropriate vaccine production strain. However, the use of cell culture can significantly accelerate the time to last dose. The markedly shorter time to production of last dose can be attributed to speed with which the cells required to produce virus can be scaled up geometrically from abundant frozen stocks (to the limit of the manufacturing capacity). In contrast, embryonated eggs are often in limited supply, especially under pandemic conditions, and can only be increased by acquiring more freshly laid eggs. For mid-level developing countries in particular, cell culture production might also be more efficient, considering the difficulty in producing sterile embryonated chicken eggs.

Mammalian cell culture techniques are used already to make a variety of human and veterinary vaccines and biologic therapeutic agents, and they have the capability to offer a predictable, rapid, and responsive method for production of well-tolerated and effective vaccines. And as was discussed in Chapter 3, other steps in the production process—development of an optimized seed strain, preparation of potency reagents, sterility testing, and fill-finish—will still have to be addressed to alleviate potential bottlenecks.

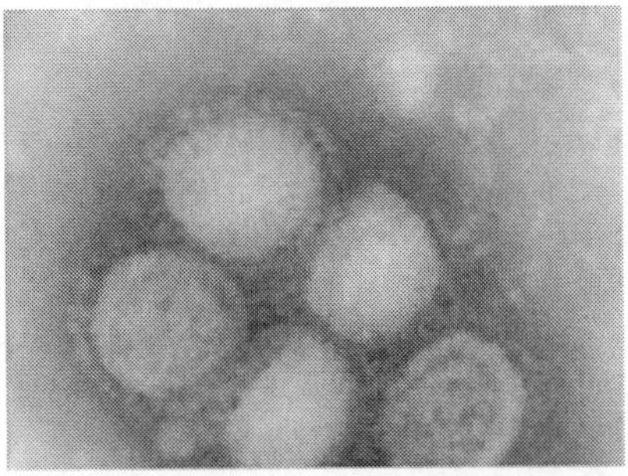

Producing influenza vaccines in cell culture is expected to shorten the timeline for the availability of the first doses of inactivated vaccine (second line) when compared to the WHO's prediction for the production of inactivated vaccine in eggs (top line); the time to release of the final doses will depend on the manufacturing capacity. Improving the initial steps to prepare, verify, and distribute vaccine strain to manufacturers and to optimize the seed virus can also be accelerated when vaccines are made in cell culture; the effects of those additional changes are shown in the third line. However, because of the accelerated manufacturing schedule, the availability of potency reagents for release testing of inactivated vaccines will become rate-limiting (orange arrow). Based on WHO predictions, potency reagents might not be available until six weeks after they were needed for final manufacturing and release.

Figure 4-1. Production Timelines for Egg and Cell Culture Inactivated Vaccines

The methods for using mammalian cell culture to produce vaccines in general—and influenza vaccines in particular—are well developed, and at least two companies have used cell culture to produce influenza vaccines that have received regulatory clearance in Europe. The majority of companies that have used or are developing cell culture methods for influenza vaccine production rely on continuous mammalian kidney cell lines, as the vehicle for producing vaccines.The main components of a mammalian cell-based influenza vaccine production system are:

- Selection of a mammalian cell line that is well-defined from a safety perspective and that is particularly suited to high-yield production of the vaccine antigen. Once the cell line is defined and characterized, it can be used for production of influenza vaccine year after year.
- Selection of an influenza seed virus that can grow to high levels in the production cell line.The seed virus would have to be antigenically matched to a given year's circulating influenza virus strain, as derived by forming reassortants between the pandemic strain and viruses known to replicate efficiently in cell culture
- Scale-up of the cell culture (and production) in a large-scale bioreactor, using defined growth medium.
- Harvesting of the virus, and subsequent processing, treatment and purification to yield bulk vaccine ready for finishing into final containers (syringes, vials, etc.) These latter steps will differ depending on whether the vaccine is to be composed of inactivated or live attenuated virus.

The basic production process is straightforward. Mammalian cells are treated with the enzyme trypsin to create a cell suspension, which is then introduced into a bioreactor (as large as 6000 liters) that allows a dramatic expansion of cell numbers. When the desired number of cells is reached, the seed strain of virus is introduced into the bioreactor, and the virus infects and replicates in the cells,The virus particles are then harvested, inactivated (except in the case of live attenuated vaccines) and purified using specially designed methods. Once this bulk vaccine is tested for concentration of antigen (potency testing for killed virus vaccine or plaque assays for LAIV) and for the absence of biological contaminants in sterility tests, it is shipped to a fill-finish facility for final preparation in individual or multipack dosage forms.

Several current vaccine manufacturers and biotechnology companies are developing technology to produce influenza vaccines using mammalian cell culture. For example, Baxter International used mammalian kidney cells to produce its 2009-H1 N1 pandemic influenza vaccine that was approved in Europe on October 6, 2009, while Novartis used a different line of mammalian kidney cells to produce its 2009-H1 N1 pandemic influenza vaccine approved in Europe on November 5, 2009. However, current capacity in the United States is inadequate to supply the quantities of cell culture-produced vaccine, especially inactivated vaccine, needed to immunize the entire population in the case of a pandemic.

4-1. Estimating the Production Capacity Needs to Cover the US Population

Vaccination of about 80% of the total US population as soon as possible after an influenza pandemic is declared—certainly before a second wave of infection begins—is the conventional goal for vaccine makers during a pandemic. That means providing about 240 million doses (Md) within one to two months after the first doses of vaccine are delivered—translating into 30 to 60 Md/week. In comparison, in 2009-2010, less than half of the desired number of doses, mostly killed, egg-based vaccine, were provided to the US population in the first three months after the first doses were delivered in early October, an average rate of about 10 Md/week.

Many variables affect the estimates of whether desired rates can be achieved: the virus yields (from eggs or cell culture), the number of manufacturers and their facilities (including the supplies of sterile embryonated eggs and the numbers and sizes of available bioreactors for cell culture), and the composition of the vaccine. For example, the yield of doses of LAIV vaccine is generally 10 to 100 times greater than for killed virus vaccine for the same amount of virus material. In addition, the number of doses of killed virus vaccine can be increased two- to ten-fold when an adjuvanted vaccine is used.

The Working Group learned that Medimmune projects that it could generate about 30 Md/week of LAIV from cell culture in four large bioreactors (G. Kemble) and that Novartis is able to produce about 10 Md/week of cell culture-derived killed vaccine (containing 3.75 ug rather than the usual 15 ug per dose, because an adjuvant was included) at its Holly Springs plant (R.Rappuoli).

Cell culture-derived vaccines and adjuvants do not yet have regulatory approval in the US and thus were not used in the US during the 2009 pandemic. However, these numbers indicate how a well-planned effort to use cell culture, LAIV, and adjuvants—together with some expansion in manufacturing capacity—could dramatically reduce the time required to provide 240 Md to the US population to one to two months.

Advantages of Producing Influenza Vaccine Using Mammalian Cell Culture

Using mammalian cell culture systems for producing influenza vaccine has several advantages over egg-based prod uction.The list of advantages includes:

- **Pre-production preparedness.** The appropriate mammalian cell lines can be stored in freezers and readied in a matter of days or weeks for large-scale production demands. In contrast, egg- based production requires secure supplies of pathogen-free, embryonated eggs, and it usually takes four to six months to generate the necessary supply of eggs from biosecure chicken flocks to meet the demands associated with either seasonal or pandemic influenza.
- **Yield and scale.** Mammalian cell lines are selected for rapid growth and production of high titers of virus, and scaling is a matter of growing more cells in bioreactors. One of the advantages of using cells to produce vaccine is that cells grow exponentially, allowing for the rapid expansion of the production substrate into large bioreactor volumes. In addition, these bioreactors can be used multiple times. Together, this allows for a relatively rapid and consistent scale-up of production, compared to what is achievable using chicken eggs.
- **Faster time to last dose.** Although it is possible to eliminate some time from the start of production to first dose using cell culture, the ability to more rapidly scale up production of virus in cell culture translates into a real benefit in terms of time required for the production of the so-called last dose, the amount needed to potentially immunize the entire population.
- **Simplified preparation and higher initial purity.** Harvesting vaccine virus particles from mammalian cell bioreactors is simpler than the methods used for sterile harvest of chicken egg allantoic

fluid. In addition, the subsequent purification of the virus yields a product of higher purity, free of contamination with egg-based allergens that can trigger hypersensitivity responses in susceptible individuals.

Barriers Impeding Influenza Vaccine Production Using Mammalian Cell Culture

The use of mammalian cell culture to produce influenza vaccines is not free of its own set of problems impeding adoption. These include:

- **Capacity.** Although vaccine production in cell culture is more readily scaled up than an egg- based process, there is still insufficient capacity at present to meet future demands in a pandemic with cell culture-based inactivated vaccine. A careful assessment of the difference between current capacity for cell culture-based production and the needed capacity to meet national demand fora pandemic inactivated influenza vaccine is required.The increase in capacity would involve the construction of facilities for additional bulk production and subsequent steps in manufacturing, as well as more efficient and flexible use of these facilities. Capacity issues would be greatly reduced if cell culture systems were also used to make LAIV vaccines, which are many-fold more potent than inactivated virus vaccine.
- **Construction costs.** The enormous expense for plant construction and validation for use as a biologics production facility poses a major problem. Novartis spent over $1 billion to construct its new large-scale cell culture-based influenza vaccine manufacturing facility in Holly Springs, NC, with the Department of Health and Human Services (HHS) contributing $487 million, or 40%, of the construction and validation costs. New plant construction, including validation and regulatory approval, takes three to four years to complete. It may be possible, however, to use existing facilities to produce virus for vaccine preparation under the appropriate biocontainment requirements in the event of an influenza pandemic.
- **Additional costs.** In any given year, a vaccine production facility may remain unused for six months in the absence of demand for a pandemic influenza vaccine, since it would be used only for seasonal

vaccine. However, preparedness for production of pandemic influenza vaccines would require maintaining trained crews to operate the cell culture production system, a significant operational cost that no company would be willing to bear. In addition, there is the "opportunity cost"of investing in plant construction and necessary research and development activities that few companies are willing to bear given the low margin nature of the influenza vaccine business. Some of these difficulties would be obviated if the facilities could be used for purposes other than production of cell-based influenza vaccines.

RECOMMENDATION 4-1. UNDERSTAND AVAILABLE CAPACITY FOR CELL CULTURE PRODUCTION AND DEVELOP INCENTIVES TO EXPAND CAPACITY

HHS, the Department of Homeland Security (DHS), and BARDA should commission a 6-month study in close collaboration with industry to determine the Nation's needs and capacity for cell culture-based production of pandemic influenza vaccine, and to develop a set of economic incentives that would catalyze the development of new influenza vaccines made in cell culture systems. Such incentives might include rapid depreciation of physical plant costs; research contracts; guaranteed purchases; cost-sharing during idle times in production plants; and construction subsidies. This study should also focus both on new capacity and the potential to utilize existing production facilities now dedicated to producing other biologicals in cell culture systems. Finally, the study should carefully consider the balance between the investment needed to increase cell culture production capacity and the possibility that novel recombinant technologies might become available soon enough to substantially diminish the need for the increased capacity required to cope with another influenza pandemic.

- **New seed viruses and potency assay reagents.** Currently, seed viruses are optimized for production of virus in chicken eggs, so it is likely that new virus backbones will be required for inactivated virus vaccines adapted to growth in mammalian cell culture. The LAIV backbone remains the same because of its attenuating characteristics but some minor modifications may enhance cell culture growth. These improvements will demand additional research and development.

Some work may also be needed to optimize the production of potency reagents specifically for vaccine antigens produced in mammalian cell culture.

RECOMMENDATION 4-2. DEVELOP OPTIMIZED SEED VIRUSES AND POTENCY ASSAYS

NIAI D and BARDA should issue a 2-year contract to develop new vaccine backbones to create seed viruses optimized for rapid growth in mammalian cell culture.

- **Regulatory uncertainty and expense.** Though two pandemic influenza vaccines (against H1N1 and a potential pandemic strain) produced in cell culture have been approved by European regulatory agencies, the Food and Drug Administration (FDA) has yet to approve an influenza vaccine produced in cell culture for use in the United States. However, on March 2, 2010, the FDA issued a final guidance document whose intent is to reduce the uncertainty surrounding the regulatory pathway for influenza vaccines produced using cell culture.[9] FDA scientists spent more than a decade conducting the research required for the document, as well as consulting with other scientists, the vaccine industry, and the public about it. In addition to providing advice to manufacturers about the scientific principles of cell substrate development, the guidance describes tests that may be used to evaluate cell substrates intended for use in viral vaccine production.

Live Attenuated Influenza Vaccine

LAIV vaccines appear to induce a potentially more effective immune response than do the comparable inactivated vaccines, especially when the vaccine recipient is"naïve"or has limited prior infections with influenza. For example, data from recent studies comparing the efficacy of inactivated influenza vaccine and LAIV vaccine in protecting children six to 59 months of age found that there were 54.9% fewer cases of confirmed influenza in the group receiving LAIV vaccine than in the group receiving inactivated virus vaccine. Superior protection against viruses that had drifted antigenically during influenza season was also seen with LAIV vaccine than with inactivated virus vaccine.[10]

RECOMMENDATION 4-3. INVESTIGATE THE IMMUNE RESPONSE TO LAIV

NIAID should increase funding for basic academic research to develop an understanding of the human immune response to LAIV vaccines and to conduct a thorough, in-depth analysis of the mechanisms that produce influenza immunity in humans. The goal of this research should be both to improve the fundamental understanding of how the human immune system responds to influenza virus and to develop new potency reagents and in vitro assays that correlate with protective immunogenicity, particularly for LAIV vaccines. Collaboration with Medlmmune, the sole commercial producer of the LAIV vaccine, would be required for some of this work.

Because LAIV vaccines may be able to trigger a more effective immune response than inactivated virus vaccines, production capacity demands in the event of a pandemic would be lower if the majority of vaccine production was devoted to LAIVvaccines. There will, however, continue to be a need to produce inactive virus vaccine because LAIV is not recommended for certain individuals such as infants and those with compromised immunity. In addition, the immunological basis of the clinical protection afforded by LAIV vaccines is not fully understood.

The FDA requires that LAIV vaccines produced in mammalian cells be shown, through an extensive efficacy trial, to be as effective as LAIV vaccines currently produced in embryonated chicken eggs; the cost of such studies typically range from $50 million to as much as $100 million.

RECOMMENDATION 4-4. SUPPORT LAIV CLINICAL TRIALS

HHS and BARDA should facilitate and share the costs of conducting the necessary clinical trials to license LAIV vaccines produced in cell culture and to generate the correlative data that will enable future LAIV vaccines to be approved for use in the same simplified manner that seasonal influenza vaccines produced in chicken eggs are today.

This cost is a major barrier to the more widespread development of LAIVs produced in mammalian cell culture, whether for seasonal or pandemic influenza.

Use of cell culture to grow cold-adapted, heat-sensitive strains of influenza virus for preparation of LAIV vaccines would have special value for shortening the time line, because viral backbones needed to generate seed stocks with appropriate properties are already available (to hasten the time to first doses) and because 50- to 100-fold less virus is generally required for an effective dose of vaccine (accelerating the time of last doses). In addition, the amount of material in LAIV vaccines is monitored by tests for infectious virus, not by potency tests, eliminating the possibility that the time course of production could be prolonged by the difficulty of preparing reagents for potency testing. However, increased production of LAIV vaccine in cell culture will not occur until clinical studies have been performed with vaccine made using this method and the vaccine has been tested in age groups for which LAIV is not currently approved.

V. Recombinant Influenza Vaccines

Section Summary

The greatest potential for substantially shortening the time and increasing the reliability of influenza vaccine production lies in the use of recombinant DNA technologies. However, as for the proposal to transition from egg-based to cell-based methods of vaccine production, there are economic barriers and regulatory uncertainties, as well as inherent biological uncertainties that are impeding the full development of these technologies. All of these uncertainties require careful definition.The economic and regulatory hurdles may require the Federal Government to provide novel incentives and pathways for development.

Production of Recombinant DNA-Based Vaccines

Today's influenza vaccines are made from whole viruses, which are strong stimulants of the immune system but are complex mixtures of materials. Egg-based products also contain potentially allergenic proteins from chicken eggs.

Fortunately, growing influenza viruses in chicken eggs or in mammalian cells in culture are not the only two methods available for making influenza vaccines. Using modern molecular technologies, a number of companies are developing what are known as recombinant vaccines—vaccines containing viral proteins synthesized under the direction of molecularly cloned viral genes and expressed in and purified from bacterial, yeast, insect, plant, or mammalian cells.

Some of the new vaccines on the market for viruses such as human papilloma and hepatitis B viruses are recombinant vaccines. Such vaccines are considered by many to be the wave of the future, but there are obstacles that must be overcome before the vaccine industry will shift from existing technologies to recombinant DNA-based technologies to replace existing vaccines. For example, as with any entirely new vaccine, recombinant vaccines require long programs of testing to establish their efficacy and safety. In addition, pure proteins often do not stimulate effective immunity and may have to be aggregated into virus-like particles and/or formulated with adjuvants to elicit protective immunity. Finally, the cost of developing such a product is an economic challenge, even for large companies.

To make recombinant influenza virus vaccines, viral genes encoding the new variant proteins must be cloned into expression vectors, most commonly viruses that infect cells of higher organisms (mammalian, insect, or plant cells) or plasmids that can replicate in bacteria or yeast. The primary goal is generally to produce large amounts of HA and other virus proteins, either as part of a virus-like particle (VLP) or as a soluble protein. In either case, proper folding of the protein will likely be needed for vaccine recipients to produce an immune response that is protective against subsequent infection by the virus. Also in development are VLPs linked to DNA sequences, which act as a built-in adjuvant, or soluble hemagglutinin protein linked to bacterial flagellin protein, which also acts as an adjuvant.Table 5-1 lists recombinant influenza vaccines being developed.

These recombinant influenza vaccines hold the promise of:

- **shortening the time to first dose of vaccine** following the identification of a novel strain of influenza virus. As illustrated in Figure 5-1, recombinant vaccines would eliminate the time now required to prepare and optimize vaccine seed stocks of virus, since production would depend instead upon molecular cloning of the viral HA gene (and perhaps other genes) from the isolated pandemic virus.

If preparation of potency reagents can be accelerated, the first doses of vaccine could be available in less than ten weeks.

- **producing larger volumes of vaccine** in any given timeframe resulting from the ability to use high-capacity platforms such as bioreactors or plants. Scaled-up production of recombinant vaccines should permit delivery of all needed doses—estimated to be in the range of 250 million—in another 4 to 6 weeks after the first doses, provided that the fill-finish process does not prove to be a bottleneck.
- **establishing extensive surge capacity** as a result of the nature of the production process, which can be readily scaled-up to meet extraordinary demands.
- **using the platform to produce other products** when it is not being used for influenza vaccine. For example, other recombinant products for use as vaccines or biological therapies might be made in the same facilities, given regulatory clearance.
- **reducing lot-to-lot variability** and the level of effort necessary for quality assurance. Recombinant procedures, in general, are more readily regularized and monitored than production of virus in eggs or mammalian cells.
- **lowering the cost of goods** relative to current production technologies. Recombinant methods are in general less expensive means of production and less subject to unexpected variations in efficiency.
- **transferring the technology to other countries,** thereby enhancing self-sufficiency of the global community and reducing political pressure on the United States to assure influenza vaccine supply for the rest of the world. Such methods have already been used to make hepatitis B vaccines in developing countries and that success should be replicable with recombinant influenza vaccines.
- **platform flexibility,** since recombinant methods can be used to design more potent HA and other antigens that might be effective for more than a single influenza season or against future pandemics, as discussed further in Chapter 7.

Table 5-1. Examples of Recombinant Influenza Vaccines in Clinical Development

Vaccine/ Manufacturer	Type	Mode of Preparation	Adjuvant	Developmental/ Regulatory Status
FluBlok®(seasonal influenza)/Protein Sciences	Soluble protein (HA), Trivalent (3 strains)	Insect cell culture/ baculovirus	None	Biological License Application Pending
PanBlock® (seasonal influenza)/ Protein Sciences	Soluble protein (HA)	Insect cell culture/ baculovirus	None Inulin, GLA being evaluated)	Clinical Trials
Influenza/ Novavax	VLP (HA, N, and M)	Insect cell culture/ baculovirus	None	Clinical Trials
Pandemic & Seasonal Influenza/ Medicago	VLP (HA and N)	Plant cell culture	None	Preclinical
Seasonal and Pandemic Influenza/ VaxInnate	Soluble human and avian protein (HA)	E. coli	Flagellin	Preclinical
Universal Influenza/ Dynavax	Soluble protein (NP, M2e)	E. coli	CpG	Preclinical
Pandemic & Seasonal Influenza/ Lentigen	VLP (HA and N)	Human cell culture/ lentivirus	None	Preclinical

VLP=virus-like particle; HA=hemagglutinin; N=neuraminidase; NP=influenza nuclear protein; M=influenza matrix protein; M2e=influenza integral membrane protein; GLA=glycopyranosyl lipid adjuvant; CpG=synthetic oligonucleotide adjuvant

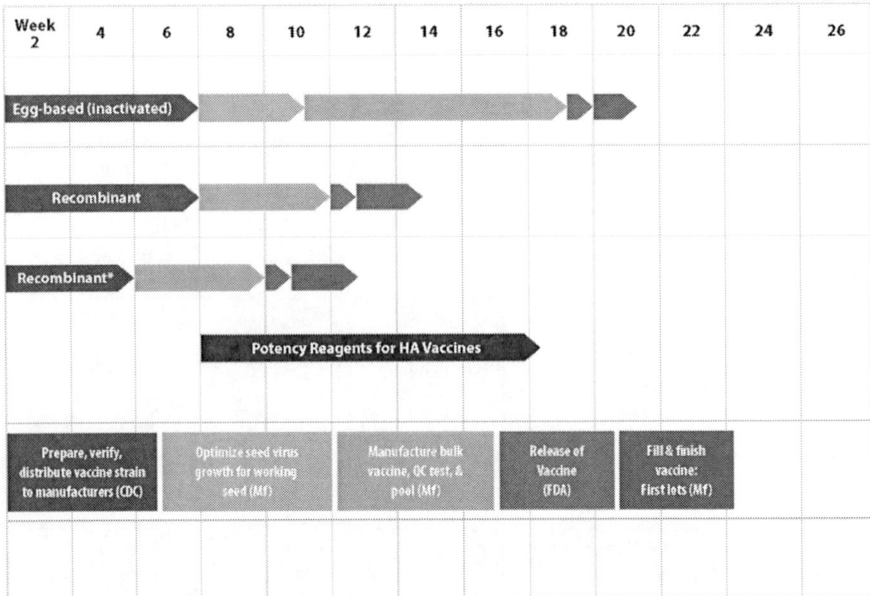

*Assumes an additional reduction time if the HA gene is cloned for possible vaccine production immediately after a novel virus is identified as causing human infection but before the virus is confirmed as a pandemic threat.

Using recombinant technology to make influenza vaccines is predicted to have a significant effect on the timeline for vaccine production (second and third lines) compared to the WHO's prediction for the production of inactivated vaccine in eggs (top line). Because there is no need with recombinant technology to create a vaccine seed virus, the process can begin as soon as the CDC has sequenced the new HA gene designated for production of pandemic influenza vaccine. Since manufacturing is readily scaled up, the time to availability of initial doses is reduced from the 20 weeks estimated for egg-based killed virus vaccine to about 12 weeks or less. To take advantage of this accelerated time line, an alternative to radial immunodiffusion with newly generated antiserum for measuring HA content as an assay of potency will be essential. The figure illustrates the time to availability of the first vaccine doses; the time to release of final doses will depend on the manufacturing capacity.

Figure 5-1 Production Timelines for Egg-based Inactivated and HA Recombinant Vaccines

Experience with Recombinant Vaccines

The majority of vaccines currently available for immunization of human beings against viral pathogens are composed of killed or live attenuated viruses, but effective recombinant vaccines against hepatitis B and human papilloma viruses (HBV and HPV) have been developed, approved, and widely used. These vaccines are manufactured by gene expression in budding yeast (Gardisil and Recombivax), mammalian cells (Energix-B), or insect cells (Cervarix). In the case of Cervarix, insect cell lines are infected with baculovirus containing a gene encoding an HPV protein, with the protein secreted into the culture medium; the vaccine protein assembles spontaneously into a VLP (virus-like particle), which increases its immunogenicity.The virus surface protein used in the HBV vaccine produced in yeast also assembles into a VLP.

Influenza vaccine antigens can also be expressed in recombinant systems, either as soluble proteins or as VLPs. Both Protein Sciences Corp. and Novavax are testing recombinant influenza vaccines. Protein Science's FluBlok, a seasonal influenza vaccine composed of purified recombinant HA antigens produced in a baculovirus cell culture system, is currently under review for licensing at the FDA. Phase III clinical trials suggest that FluBlok may be more effective than standard influenza vaccine in triggering an HA antibody response equal to that produced by standard vaccine in people over 65, a population that accounts for over 90% of influenza-related deaths in most years. The company's PanBlok, a pandemic influenza vaccine candidate comprising purified recombinant HA from the H5N1 avian influenza virus, is in Phase II clinical trials. Novavax's recombinant pandemic influenza vaccine, this one designed to protect against the 2009 H1 N1 influenza virus, consists of VLPs composed of HA and N produced in a baculovirus cell culture system.This vaccine is currently in Phase II trials. The company's seasonal influenza vaccine, also consisting of recombinant antigens produced in baculovirus cell culture, is in Phase Ila clinical trials.

One of the major advantages of using eukaryotic cells—those of higher organisms, including mammals—to produce viral proteins for vaccines is that they generate proteins that are more likely to be properly folded and modified with the proper sugar molecules than are proteins produced in bacterial expression systems. Although the pattern of glycosylation (the arrangement of sugars on a protein) obtained using insect cells may differ from that in mammalian or avian cells, influenza proteins produced with baculovirus vectors in insect cells have proven to be immunogenic and to provide protection against influenza in the widely used ferret challenge model[11 12]. These proteins have also been able to trigger antibody production against the recombinant proteins in human clinical trial subjects.[13]

It is possible that recombinant vaccines will not trigger an immune response strong enough to protect against infection. In such cases, it is likely that adjuvant will be needed to overcome that limitation. (See Chapter 6 for a discussion of adjuvants.)

Once a recombinant influenza vaccine is established as safe and effective through clinical trials, the FDA will likely approve future recombinant vaccines made using the same expression system by a mechanism similar to the regulatory process now used to approve new seasonal influenza vaccines containing different strains of virus.

Taking the Initiative

Despite their potential advantages, recombinant influenza vaccines—with the possible exception of Protein Sciences'Flu Blok which is currently under review by the FDA—will likely take several years, and possibly more than a decade, to reach the market. This is especially true without the direct involvement of and active management by the Federal Government.

Recommendation 5-1. Launch a 3-by-3 Recombinant Influenza Vaccine Initiative

The working group recommends that the Federal Government establish a recombinant influenza vaccine initiative (see box below for details), constituted under the authority of the Assistant Secretary for Preparedness and Response (ASPR) at HHS, with a goal of advancing at least three recombinant influenza vaccines that are suitable for use against seasonal or pandemic influenza to proof-of-concept trials within three years.This initiative should be overseen by a group comprised of representatives from BARDA, FDA, NIAID, and CDC, reporting to the ASPR, with input from the relevant components of DOD and DHS.

While there are ongoing efforts to develop recombinant influenza vaccines (predominantly by biotechnology companies), the seasonal vaccine market is currently fully saturated with effective and modestly priced vaccines; hence the economic incentives that would normally drive the application of novel technologies are not present. PCAST believes the Federal Government should take a number of steps to provide clear signals that endorse financial and regulatory support to the industry, and to the investment, public health, and medical communities, so that they are more likely to undertake the efforts necessary to bring these products to market for seasonal influenza, and to ensure that these technologies will be available to produce influenza vaccines during a pandemic.

5-1. Elements of a Recombinant Influenza Vaccine Initiative

A recombinant influenza vaccine initiative will consist of several components, each of which will require action on the part of HHS to achieve the initiative's goal of advancing candidate vaccines to proof-of-concept trials within the next three years. In order to achieve this goal, HHS should:

1. Engage representatives from industry and the investment community in the design and management of the initiative. HHS has limited experience managing complex external research and development projects. Moreover, the biotechnology and pharmaceutical industries operate in a complex marketplace. It is therefore important that the Federal Government engage these communities in the design and execution of the initiative. As a starting point, the Federal Government should publish a roadmap of the steps it is taking to accelerate the development of recombinant influenza vaccines in order to ensure broad awareness and input to the design and execution of this enterprise. An advisory committee, including representatives from industry and the investment community, should be established to ensure that HHS's decisions and actions are informed by perspectives from these two stakeholders, given the importance that their actions will have on the success and sustainability of the initiative.
2. Provide clean guidance on the minimal essential attributes of a novel recombinant influenza vaccine, and capture these attributes in a target product profile. In consultation with stakeholders in the Federal Government, industry, and the medical and public health communities, the Federal Government should define the minimal attributes of the

desired vaccine, for both seasonal and pandemic uses, including criteria for: formulation, presentation, storage and administration, safety, immunogenicity and efficacy. This guidance should be updated as new tools for validation (e.g., potency assays, immune correlates) are identified.

3. Provide clean guidance on the minimal essential attributes of a novel recombinant influenza vaccine, and capture these attributes in a target product profile. In consultation with stakeholders in the Federal Government, industry, and the medical and public health communities, the Federal Government should define the minimal attributes of the desired vaccine, for both seasonal and pandemic uses, including criteria for: formulation, presentation, storage and administration, safety, immunogenicity and efficacy. This guidance should be updated as new tools for validation (e.g., potency assays, immune correlates) are identified.
4. Provide clear guidance on the required timeline for production of the first doses of pandemic vaccine and the number of doses that must be produced within a window of time. The principal benefit of a recombinant influenza vaccine in the context of pandemic planning is the speed of production of the first doses of vaccine and scale-up of manufacturing.The minimum requirements for the time to first dose and the time to production of sufficient doses for the United States population should be defined at the outset of this effort, and should be driven by what is necessary to ensure an effective pandemic response, rather than what is thought to be possible with today's technologies.
5. Establish a regulatory pathway for the review and approval of this platform for seasonal influenza, and the regulatory requirements for a pandemic vaccine produced on this platform. There is currently great uncertainty about the regulatory pathway for recombinant influenza vaccines. To focus current product development efforts and provide a level of certainty to the biotechnology and investment communities, it is essential that the Federal Government define the regulatory pathway for these new technologies for seasonal influenza, and the criteria that will be applied in the context of a pandemic, for platforms that have been approved for the production of a seasonal vaccine.
6. Develop an investment strategy that allows co-financing of promising vaccine production platforms, and create downstream incentives for products that meet the target product profile and production criteria.To advance promising technologies, and to incentivize additional external

investment, the Federal Government may need to make direct investments in companies with promising platforms to push them through clinical development and eventual licensure for seasonal influenza. Making this investment may necessitate co-financing with venture capital firms and other investors; it may also require flexibility in the terms of such investments. Investing in recombinant vaccines may also require the establishment of additional downstream incentives such as advance market commitments or prizes, and allowance for companies to use the technologies and platforms to produce products for other conditions, including those that provide greater profit incentive and more certainty of demand.

7. Establish Federal policy for the use of recombinant influenza vaccines in seasonal influenza campaigns and during a pandemic, once they have been proven to be safe and efficacious. Given the barriers to entry of a novel vaccine into the mature influenza vaccine market, the Federal Government should make it clear that recombinant vaccines will eventually comprise a portion of the Federal tender for seasonal influenza vaccines, and that appropriate technical platforms are part of a long-term strategy for pandemic preparedness.This will serve as an incentive for manufacturers, and should also serve to make their technologies more attractive to the investment community.

VI. Adjuvants

Section Summary

Adjuvants are substances or mixtures of substances added to a vaccine to enhance the immunological response to the vaccine. Although their use in influenza vaccines has been limited to date, adjuvants have a long history of safe and effective use in human vaccines. Their primary use in vaccines has been to boost the immune response to vaccination among the elderly and other individuals with health conditions that suppress the normal immune response; broaden the immune response to a vaccine to provide better protection against a virus if it mutates; prolong the duration of immunity; and stretch the supply of vaccine when supplies are tight. Because of these benefits, adjuvants should have an important role to play in meeting the Nation's demand for influenza vaccine during a pandemic, but scientific and regulatory barriers present significant obstacles that can be addressed through additional research and guidance from the FDA.

Regardless of how influenza vaccine is produced, whether in eggs, cell culture, or by recombinant methods, adjuvants are a key component to improving how pandemics can be dealt with in the future. Adjuvants are components that boost vaccine potency, so that the vaccines can induce an effective immune response with lower doses of vaccine protein. Adopting adjuvants, several of which are already components in approved vaccines, including certain influenza vaccines used in Europe, can be both a mid- and long-term solution to boosting influenza vaccine supply. Adjuvants can be stockpiled in large amounts, and there is no need to vary adjuvant composition from one pandemic strain to the next. In addition, adjuvants can increase the breadth of the immune response to afford protection against both the targeted vaccine strain as well as related strains.

Adjuvants have a long history of safe and effective use in human vaccines, but their use in influenza vaccines has been limited. This chapter will discuss how adjuvants might fit into a national pandemic influenza strategy and examine steps that the Federal Government can take to facilitate the use of adjuvanted influenza vaccines.

What Is an Adjuvant and Why Are Adjuvants Added to Vaccines?

An adjuvant is a substance or mixture of substances added to a vaccine to enhance the immune response to the vaccine. Examples of adjuvants used today in human viral vaccines, or under development for future use, include alum (aluminum hydroxide), oil-and-water emulsions, particulates, microbial and plant derivatives, and so-called Toll-like receptor (TLR)-related molecules designed to stimulate the Toll-like receptors, which are involved in triggering an immune response.

There are four potential benefits to using adjuvants to improve vaccines:

- **to boost the immune response** in certain age groups (particularly the elderly) or in people with underlying health conditions who cannot mount an adequate immune response to a vaccine made without adjuvant;

- **to broaden the immune response** to a vaccine to provide better protection that can accommodate the genetic diversity of influenza viruses;
- **to prolong the duration of immunity** and improve immunological memory that can protect against infection for years; and
- **to increase or stretch the vaccine supply** if it is limited.

Antigens vary in their physical, biological and immunogenic properties and may have different needs for help from an adjuvant. Successful vaccine development requires knowing which adjuvants to use based on the antigen and the desired immune response, as well as knowing how to formulate adjuvants and antigens to achieve stable, safe, and immunogenic vaccines. For some vaccines, such as those produced by recombinant methods (see Chapter 5), adjuvants may prove to be critical for triggering a sufficient immune response following vaccination. By stretching a limited vaccine supply, addition of adjuvants can shorten the time between provision of the first and last doses by several weeks. In addition, because some adjuvants cost less than the viral materials in killed vaccines, regardless of whether the virus is produced in an egg-based or cell culture system, adjuvant use can reduce the cost of the final vaccine by increasing the number of doses that can be prepared from viral materials. This could have especially important implications for provision of a pandemic vaccines to poor countries.

Selection of appropriate adjuvants, from the limited number available, is based on the nature of the antigen and immune response desired. For a long lasting immune response, adjuvants that stimulate T cell responses are desired. However, T cell responses are not optimally induced by emulsions or alum, particularly when used with purified recombinant proteins that do not trigger activity via TLRs on immune cells. Vaccines produced from virus grown in chicken eggs or cell culture contain variable amounts of viral RNA, which can be a natural adjuvant and is not present in vaccines composed of recombinant proteins. The mechanisms by which adjuvants boost the immune response are understood in some cases, but less so for most adjuvants.

No human influenza vaccines licensed in the United States use an adjuvant, though adjuvanted influenza vaccines are approved for human use in Europe.

Recommendation 6-1. Improve Basic Knowledge about Adjuvant Immunology

The National Institute of Allergy and Infectious Diseases (NIAID) should increase funding for basic research on immunology with the goal of understanding how adjuvants improve the body's response to vaccination, particularly in the context of recombinant vaccine candidates. Not only will such research clarify the basic mechanisms by which adjuvants work, but it should also lead to more potent vaccines that are safe and well-tolerated. This avenue of research could also alleviate perceived safety concerns among some segments of the public. It will be important to include early stage clinical studies as an essential part of the research.

Until recently, alum was the only adjuvant approved for use in human vaccines, and in fact, the FDA does not approve adjuvants per se, but does approve specific adjuvant-vaccine combinations. Gardasil, the first HPV vaccine licensed in the United States, uses alum as its adjuvant. In late 2009, the FDA approved the use of ASO4, a new adjuvant composed of alum and a bacterial product known as monophosphoryl lipid A (MPL), as components of Cervarix, the second vaccine licensed to prevent HPV infection.

Recommendation 6-2. Develop Adjuvant Guidance Document

Adjuvants can be an important mid-term solution to vaccine supply and will be an essential component to a long term solution of developing recombinant protein based influenza vaccines.The FDA should develop and issue a guidance document that defines a clear regulatory pathway for the approval of adjuvants for use in human vaccines, including those for seasonal and pandemic influenza.This guidance document should define the goals for adjuvant use (i.e., dose sparing, boosting efficacy in the elderly), specify rational endpoints for clinical trials, and stipulate safety criteria. Because the safety and efficacy of adjuvants can only be evaluated in the context of the final vaccine product, the current practice of approving final products, as opposed to adjuvants alone, is a rational one.

In the event of a declared emergency, the FDA can approve the use of adjuvanted vaccine under an Emergency Use Authorization, and during the 2009 H1 N1 pandemic, HHS purchased supplies of adjuvant as a contingency, although adjuvanted vaccine was not used.

Adjuvant Candidates for Influenza Vaccines

The most commonly used adjuvant formulations include alum, which helps promote antibody responses for many vaccines. Alum is used in vaccines because of its long-term safety record and the ease with which it can be formulated with vaccine antigen. However, alum has not proven to be effective for influenza vaccines. For influenza vaccines, developers are focusing on two types of adjuvants: emulsions (oil in water) and TLR-related molecules. For next generation vaccines, there will be several adjuvant options available that should be explored.

Emulsions. These are the most widely use adjuvants for influenza vaccines. Indeed, there is an extensive history of using vaccines containing oil. Ninety years ago, the United States military developed typhoid vaccines that were mixed with oil with the intent of doing what vaccine manufacturers are still striving for today—decreasing the amount of vaccine antigen needed for protection, and decreasing the number of immunizations required for protection.The next generation of oil-based adjuvants were water-in-oil emulsions, used in a licensed influenza vaccine in the United Kingdom in the 1960s. Although the overall safety profile for this vaccine was excellent, the occurrence of local inflammatory responses in some patients led to withdrawal of the vaccine.

Today, three major emulsion-type adjuvants are under development.

- AS03, created by GlaxoSmithKline and contained in an influenza vaccine licensed in Europe, is a squalene-based emulsion that also contains vitamin E. Squalene is a naturally occurring chemical involved in the body's production of cholesterol and vitamin D. For commercial use, squalene is harvested primarily from shark liver oil, but also from plant vegetable oils. Vaccines containing AS03 have been evaluated in thousands of individuals, and an AS03-H5N1 influenza vaccine has been reported to be safe in both adults and children. AS03 is being developed for both seasonal and pandemic influenza vaccines, including pre-pandemic vaccines to prime individuals against H5 viruses to induce at least partial immunity against related influenza variants. The vaccine has been reported to be immunogenic, dose-sparing, and able to induce immune responses against influenza viruses in the H5 family other than the one incorporated in the vaccine. Approximately 70 million doses of AS03-containing H1N1 vaccine were distributed during the 2009 pandemic, with several million doses used in Canada and throughout the European Union (EU).

- Novartis's squalene-containing adjuvant, MF59, is licensed in Europe for use in influenza vaccines, and MF59-antigen formulations have been tested in herpes simplex virus (HSV), hepatitis B virus (HBV), and human immunodeficiency virus (HIV) vaccine candidates. Increased immunogenicity has been achieved with MF59-adjuvanted seasonal influenza vaccines in the elderly, and with MF59-adjuvanted vaccines against cytomegalovirus and HIV in young children. An estimated 45 million doses or more of Novartis's MF59-containing seasonal influenza vaccine have been administered in Europe, providing a good safety data base for MF59. During the 2009 H1N1 pandemic, approximately 70 million doses of an MF59-adjuvanted H1N1 vaccine were distributed, with an estimated 15 million doses administered in Canada and the EU.
- AF3 is a third squalene-based emulsion adjuvant, developed by Sanofi Pasteur. This adjuvant has been evaluated in a H5N1 vaccine candidate in 251 healthy adults; the vaccine was found to be adequately safe and immunogenic, and the adjuvant demonstrated both a dose sparing and immune broadening effect.

TLR-related molecules. This class of adjuvants includes the bacterial component MPL, the only TLRrelated molecule licensed for use as an adjuvant in human vaccines. MPL is a component of both HPV and HBV vaccines, although the latter is licensed only in Europe. MPL is also a component of a vaccine used to desensitize against pollen allergies, and has been demonstrated to be safe, well-tolerated, and effective. Another bacterial protein, known as flagellin, is being tested as an adjuvant in an influenza vaccine being developed by Vaxinnate. Clinical studies have demonstrated that flagellin does boost vaccine potency, but with a narrow dose range of tolerability. None of theseTLR-related adjuvants have yet been used to demonstrate dose-sparing capabilities.

RECOMMENDATION 6-3. NEW ADJUVANTS

Because adjuvants are a critical component of both mid- and long-terms solutions for improving quality and quantity of influenza vaccines, NIAID and BARDA should increase funding for the development of new adjuvants for use with influenza vaccines based on advances in understanding mechanisms of how adjuvants work. It is likely that such adjuvants will also be effective at boosting the potency of other vaccines that are important for medical countermeasures.

In addition to emphasizing development, investment in manufacturing of new adjuvants will be critical for ensuring adequate supply. Such an investment will represent eventual cost savings as needs for vaccine manufacturing capacity will be reduced as a result of including adjuvants in the final product. It is likely, too, that emulsions currently used in killed influenza vaccines can lead to a dose-sparing effect of at least 2-4 fold, which could significantly increase current supply. The role of adjuvants in enhancing potency of LAIVs is less clear, and studies should be undertaken to investigate this possibility. Because the nature of the vaccine (i.e. recombinant, killed, or attenuated virus) will directly influence the choice of adjuvants, it is increasingly important to develop a broader adjuvant pipeline. It is recommended that the FDA work closely with vaccine manufacturers to meet the goal of approving a minimum of two adjuvanted influenza vaccines in the next two years.

Adjuvants can be an important component of addressing influenza vaccine supply, particularly at the global level. In the short term, emulsions can be used to begin to address this need, as they can be produced on a large scale, have good stability, and can be combined with several of the current vaccines. However, emulsion technology itself will eventually need to be improved, as all contain shark liver oil, a non-sustainable resource. In the mid-term, improved emulsions, as well as emulsions or other formulations containing immune activators such as TLR-related molecules, are likely to be included as key components of vaccine development, but only if a clear regulatory pathway for their approval can be defined.

VII. " Universal" Influenza Vaccines

Section Summary

Influenza virus is an unusual pathogen, one that evolves regularly into new strains that avoid the protection conferred by vaccines that induced protection against strains of influenza virus circulating in prior years. As a result, each influenza season brings with it the need to prepare a new influenza vaccine against that year's crop of seasonal influenza viruses. More importantly, the same need to create a new vaccine arises when a new strain of pandemic influenza virus appears on the world stage. However, recent research raises the tantalizing possibility that there may be parts of the influenza virus that do not mutate and that could serve as the immunological basis for creating a "universal" influenza vaccine, one that would protect against both present and future strains of influenza virus.Though it is uncertain that a universal influenza vaccine is possible, the game-changing potential of such a vaccine warrants a concerted research effort supported by the Federal Government.

Life-long vaccine protection against most viral pathogens is conceptually easy to imagine. Starting with a natural strain of the virus, one makes a preparation of live, killed, or subunit viral material which, when injected into a person, provides the protection. This has worked for each of the 3 strains of poliovirus, for smallpox, mumps, measles, hepatitis B, and several other viruses. The injected preparation induces the person's immune system to make antibody proteins, which provide the first line of protection, and perhaps immune killer cells that contribute to host defenses. Life-long protection is provided because the viruses never significantly change their structure sufficiently to elude the primed immune system of the vaccinated person.

Almost all viruses for which we have long-lasting vaccine protection are viruses that have evolved for millions of years as human pathogens. Most of them infect only humans. They have developed a nonlethal relationship with humans; the viruses don't kill most infected people, although infection can be very unpleasant. We make vaccines to protect against the rare lethal consequences of infection and to minimize illnesses, but the natural relationship of the viruses to their hosts is a truce. If these viruses infected animals, they would have the chance to mutate into a different form, possibly eluding the truce with humans and becoming more lethal. However, it is hard for a virus to infect two different species efficiently because in adapting to one, it loses adaptation to the other.

For most viruses for which vaccines have been successfully created, the vaccine is either a chemically treated, non-infectious form of the virus or a live but genetically altered virus strain that grows in a vaccinated person but does not cause symptoms. Examples include polio, measles, mumps, and varicella (chicken pox) vaccines. More recently, for some viruses that have not been amenable to development of the classic forms of vaccine, vaccines containing only viral proteins have been created using recombinant DNA techniques. These recombinant vaccines are safe, because they do not start with live virus but rather consist of purified proteins made in animal or plant cells, yeast, or bacteria.

There are three viruses for which even modern protein technology has so far been unable to generate long-lasting immunity: hepatitis C virus, human immunodeficiency virus (HIV), and influenza virus. For each of these, the challenge is different, and each must be approached separately. As described in the earlier sections of this chapter, effective influenza vaccines do exist, but they are not universal; they do not protect against the virus generically but rather protect against only a very limited set of closely related influenza strains. The challenge of producing a universal influenza virus vaccine is to find a region of the virus that does not vary year to year but is both a target of antibodies and is able to induce such antibodies.

Up to now, the vaccine industry has focused on making vaccines to order for each year's expected outbreak of seasonal influenza. This works well as long the drift of virus structure is small and the forewarning is early enough to allow the slow process of vaccine production to make sufficient vaccine for the expected yearly appearance of the new strains in the late fall or winter of the year. However, there would be serious trouble if the warning is late, if a strain appears at an odd time, if a shift of viral structure has occurred, if a virulent bird strain were to adapt to humans directly, or if other imaginable events occurred to limit vaccine effectiveness. The other parts of this chapter deal with stop-gap measures that would speed up the response if any of these problems arose. However, there is another way to prepare for such eventualities: to produce a single vaccine that provided wide coverage against many if not all flu strains for a long time, maybe a lifetime, just like we do for so many other viruses. We propose to call such a vaccine a "universal vaccine".

Is a Universal Vaccine Conceivable?

When killed preparations of influenza virus are used as a vaccine, a vaccinated person produces antibodies. These antibodies bind to active virus particles of the same type and make them non-infectious, a process called virus neutralization. This reaction of antibody with virus protects a vaccinated individual against getting the symptoms of influenza disease after exposure to virus. The body's immune system, which makes antibodies, also produces a different form of immunity, one managed by so-called T cells. Vaccination may also produce a T cell response, but it is not clear whether it contributes to protection, although it is likely to help antibody production and could kill infected cells.

With influenza virus, the anti-viral antibodies react with viral HA protein. Figure 7-1 shows the structure of the portion of the HA protein that is normally found on the surface of the virus. HA is responsible for binding to the surface of an infected cell and initiating the infection of that cell. It does so by binding to a sugar called sialic acid, which is a material attached to many of the proteins found on the surface of cells. The cell is then stimulated to take the bound virus particle into its interior. (From here on, infection of the cell involves the virus taking over the RNA and protein synthetic ability of the cell and diverting these capabilities to the manufacture of new virus.) Anti-HA antibodies react with the top of the HA protein, occluding the hole at the top of HA into which the sialic acid must fit if infection is to be initiated. Like all proteins, HA is made of amino acids; the antibodies actually bind to the amino acids lining the hole.

Influenza virus can elude immune attack by mutating, which can change the amino acids around the hole. Presumably, this happens occasionally when the virus is multiplying in a human host, but these altered strains generally take a year or longer to become a dominant part of the influenza virus mixture spreading among humans.Thus, the vaccine works for about a year but by then the spreading influenza virus has a predominant structure that is resistant to the antibodies elicited by the strain of the past year. One might imagine that there could be amino acids at the top of HA that are so important to the function of the protein that they cannot be changed without compromising virus infectivity. Such amino acids could then be the target of a universal vaccine. However, no such amino acids are known; therefore, if we are to make a universal vaccine, it would seem to require a new approach.

Recent research has identified antibodies that react with another part of the HA and neutralize the virus.[14] These antibodies react with the long stem of

HA, not the top part; how they neutralize the protein and its function is unclear. HA undergoes an obligate structural alteration to get influenza virus into host cells, and the antibody is likely to interfere with the protein's molecular movement. These antibodies react with a wide range of influenza strains but not all; they are a clear starting point for development of a universal vaccine.

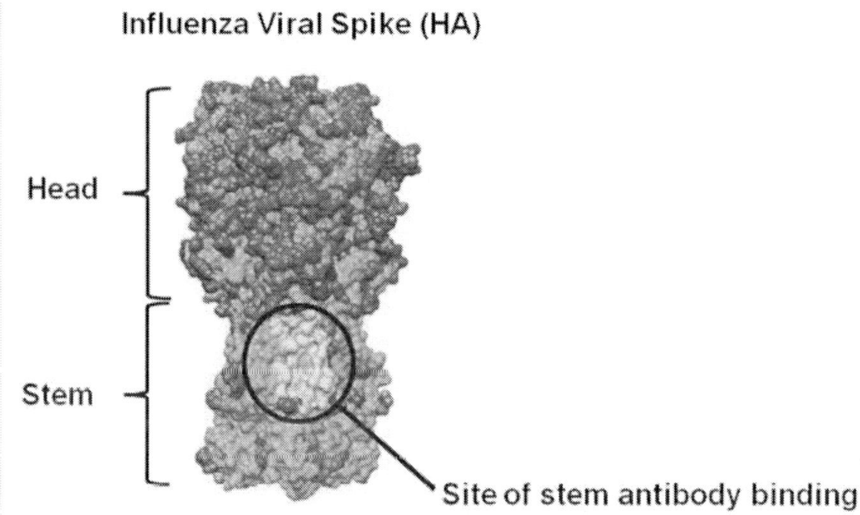

Molecular model of the part of the hemagglutinin (HA) protein that forms a "spike' on the surface of the influenza virus particle, showing the site of the highly conserved region that offers vulnerability to a "universal" vaccine. The HA spike is composed of an upper (head) and lower (stem) region, it mediates attachment and entry of influenza virus into cells of the respiratory tract; and it serves as the target for neutralizing antibodies against influenza viruses. The sites of amino acid variability among different influenza strains (red, purple, blue) and the location of the highly conserved site (yellow), the target for cross-reactive antibody against the stem portion, are highlighted.

Source: Gary Nabel, Director, Vaccine Research Center, National Institute of Allergy and Infectious Diseases, Personal Communication, May 28, 2010.

Figure 7-1. Influenza Hemagglutinin Protein

Having antibodies that neutralize a wide range of influenza virus strains is only a start toward a universal vaccine. The next step is to design an immunogen, a material that can induce people's immune system to make such antibodies. This is not an easy task, since it means making a mimic of the region of HA to which the neutralizing antibody binds. This is a very difficult design challenge; no vaccine available today involves a protein mimic of this sort.

It is possible to imagine other targets for a universal vaccine. The neuraminidase (N) protein could be a target, since it is also a target for neutralizing antibodies although the mechanism of neutralization is not certain.There is a small amount of a third protein in the virus's surface, called M2, that is needed for infection. It, too, is being developed as a target for vaccination.[15] There are others regions of proteins in the virus structure that could be targets ofT cell immunity, but they are unlikely to be universal targets because T cells recognize small fragments of viral proteins together with the highly variable host cell proteins to which they are bound. The consequence is that a vaccine stimulating T cell immunity may be effective in some people but not others.

Antibodies that neutralize many influenza strains are not only valuable for guiding immunogen design. They could, in principle, be made in large quantities using recombinant DNA technology and be delivered to protect against influenza viruses. To be protective, the antibodies themselves would have to be administered to people on a periodic basis, with that interval depending on the stability of the antibodies in the body. Antibodies are quite stable proteins in the blood, so the interval between administrations could be as long as 6 months; but this is not as convenient as the life-long protection offered by vaccines containing immunogen. Antibodies are being considered as protective materials for preventing AIDS in high risk populations, but for something as widespread as influenza virus infection, it is unclear that treatment with antibody would be cost-effective or even feasible.

However, discovery of an antibody that protects against infection should generate concentrated activity to produce an immunogen that elicits the antibody. In particular, the discovery of an antibody that protects against many influenza strains should stimulate research to mimic the surface of the influenza HA to which the antibody binds, in an effort to immunize with a mimic of the binding site. This is already under way for the antibodies that bind to the so-called "stem" region of HA.

An important question about a universal vaccine is how"universal"it is. There are multiple Type A influenza strains and also a B strain incorporated into current seasonal vaccines. Type A and B viruses might prove to be sensitive to some of the same antibodies but, more likely, each will require its own vaccine. Also, we can imagine that some improved immunogens might induce reactivity with some HA subtypes of A strains but not others. Thus, there may be a need for multiple components to make influenza vaccines that approach universality. Furthermore, if the antibodies elicited by a vaccine are highly focused on one part of the HA molecule, the virus may be able to mutate to resistance, evading the protective effects of the antibodies. Such a virus could then spread widely, making the vaccine impotent.

In truth, we have much to learn about human immunity and about how protective antibodies are elicited from the huge repertoire of antibodies that the body could make. Study of antibody production by the human immune system has been neglected by immunologists in recent times in favor of work on T cell immunity, which is thought to be the more exciting field of research today. But since antibodies seem to be the major form of protection against most viruses, with some assistance from T cells, a renewed research focus on antibody elicitation is in order.

The value of having a universal influenza vaccine would be enormous because it would be made by chemistry or by simple protein production methods, and therefore the vaccine would be scalable and storable. If it were truly universal—that is covered all of the known HA subtypes—then the likelihood of a resistant strain emerging would be slight (one might come from a strain not encountered to date in nature or from a rare recombinant between existing strains). A universal vaccine would be a "disruptive technology;" but it would reward its inventors handsomely because it would be so much preferable to the present annual race to make vaccine or the periodic race to blunt a pandemic.

RECOMMENDATION 7-1. UNIVERSAL VACCINE INITIATIVE

Because a universal vaccine would completely change the outlook on protecting the population against influenza virus infections, the Federal Government should support and encourage efforts to design a universal vaccine through various mechanisms. One is the standard mechanism of peer-reviewed grants that supports all basic health science. Imaginative ideas should be encouraged and money should be set aside for this effort. Because some ideas are further advanced, they should be supported by more targeted efforts to bring them to clinical testing. When proof of principle has been attained, the relevant agencies should encourage and, when necessary, support, commercial development. An X Prize-like competition should be considered for stimulating research on forms of a universal vaccine.

Recommendation 7-2. Basic Immunology

Although there is much to be learned yet from model organisms such as the mouse, there is insufficient research effort focused on understanding the human immune system. In particular, there should be a targeted focus on a better understanding of antibody production in human beings. The NIAID should expand and emphasize programs of support for the basic science underlying vaccine development.

VIII. A New Way of Doing business

Section Summary

In this chapter, the PCAST Influenza Vaccinology Working Group lays out a number of near-, mid-, and short- term strategies to shorten the time required to produce influenza vaccine against new pandemic influenza viruses and to reduce the risk that the Nation will be unable to respond effectively in the event of an influenza pandemic. For this effort to succeed, the Federal Government must take a mission-driven approach to reengineering the vaccine enterprise, with clear milestones and deliverables, and develop new policies, regulations, systems, and processes to support this effort.

HHS is the agency charged with protecting the Nation's health, and is best positioned to oversee this effort. Given the ambition and complexity of this undertaking, the Working Group believes that HHS should ensure that the capabilities and capacities necessary to execute this mission-driven research and development enterprise are in place. Indeed, the Working Group believes that a new way of doing business is in order, one that centralizes authority and accountability for the influenza vaccine enterprise and that can manage the complex set of short, medium, and long-term actions necessary to achieve its vaccine development and production objectives.

HHS should vest ASPR with the authority to coordinate and task its component agencies with activities necessary to support the goals of the influenza vaccine enterprise. In addition, HHS should establish a small advisory committee, comprised of representatives from the biotechnology, pharmaceutical and investment communities, to guide its engagement with industry. This committee's input should be considered seriously in all decisions and actions by the Department, given the importance of the relationship between the Federal Government and industry partners.

HHS should also establish a dedicated entity, either within the Department (for example, under BARDA) or through an external organization, such as an FFRDC or PDP, to oversee the entire portfolio of Federal investments in the influenza vaccine enterprise.

Whatever the details of this new management structure, it is essential that any planning activities for this reengineering take place with the full cooperation and participation of the private sector, that HHS work collaboratively with other federal agencies, and that the White House, most appropriately the National Security Council, assume responsibility for defining and monitoring progress towards the goals of the vaccine program. It is also important that the Federal Government's influenza vaccine efforts be aligned with changes being made to the Nation's broader medical countermeasures enterprise.

While the recent H1N1 pandemic stretched the United States Government's capabilities, it is clear that the situation could have been much worse. Taken in conjunction with the lessons learned about pandemic preparedness and the broader medical countermeasure enterprise over the past several years, the Federal Government should view this as a wake-up call and an opportunity to rethink the manner in which it prepares for pandemic influenza and other biological threats.

This chapter outlines a series of near-, mid-, and long-term strategies to shorten the timeframe to availability of sufficient influenza vaccine to protect the domestic population. For this effort to be successful, the Federal Government must take a mission-driven approach to reengineering the influenza vaccine enterprise, with clear milestones and deliverables, and develop new policies, regulations, systems, and processes to support this effort.

Assigning Responsibilities

While HHS and its component agencies (NIH, FDA, CDC, and BARDA) are responsible for the health of the Nation and medical elements of pandemic preparedness, aligning the efforts of these agencies toward a common objective can be challenging. Each agency has its own mandate and budget, as well as ongoing responsibilities and capacity limitations. Moreover, HHS has limited experience in mission- driven research and development.

In order for HHS to execute the recommendations in this chapter, it will be necessary for the Department to establish a new way of doing business. This will necessitate the centralization of authority and accountability for the influenza vaccine enterprise within the Department, and the establishment of an entity to manage the complex set of short, medium, and long-term actions necessary to achieve its vaccine development and production objectives. While HHS could establish this capacity and expertise "in house"another option is for these responsibilities to be handled through an external agent such as a Federally Funded Research and Development Center (FFRDC) or a Product Development Partnership (PDP), similar to those that have been established to coordinate and drive the development of specific countermeasures against global health threats, such as the Malaria Vaccine Initiative and theTB Alliance. This entity should oversee the breadth of activities necessary for the success of the enterprise and the portfolio companies, including horizon (technology) scanning, portfolio management, pre-clinical and clinical development, regulatory affairs, commercialization, financial management, and business development.

It is also important that HHS leverage the expertise and capacity of relevant departments and agencies across the Federal Government, including DOD, DHS, the Department of Agriculture (USDA) and the State Department, as it executes this mission. A number of attempts have been made to do this in the past, including through coordination by HHS or the White House. The lessons from these efforts should be incorporated into a management structure that places HHS in charge of this mission to protect the civilian public, but ensures that the Department is sufficiently coordinated with the other relevant components of the Federal Government. This can be accomplished by a clearly-delineated set of goals and deliverables that are developed and monitored by the White House, most appropriately by the staff of the National Security Council, in coordination with the Departmental agencies.

Recommendation 8-1. Managing a Mission-Driven Enterprise

The Administration should clearly delineate its short-, medium-, and long-term influenza vaccine development and production goals, with associated milestones and deliverables. HHS should be given responsibility for progress toward these goals and for coordinating its activities with the relevant departments and agencies that have expertise and programs relevant to influenza vaccine development and deployment. Given that the Secretary of HHS has limited authority to direct the actions of other departments such as DoD, the responsibilities of these other agencies should be made explicit by the White House.

While HHS will manage the day-to-day activities of the influenza vaccine enterprise, it is important that the Administration track progress toward its pandemic preparedness goals and the contributions of the relevant departments and agencies by establishing accountability mechanisms. The White House has traditionally played this role in policy development and execution, and the National Security Council (NSC) would be the most appropriate lead for this function.

Recommendation 8-2. Coordination of Actions Within HHS

HHS should vest ASPR with the authority to coordinate and task its component agencies with activities necessary to support the goals of the influenza vaccine enterprise. Each agency should have clearly-delineated responsibilities and deliverables that should be reflected in their respective budgets and programs, and each should be held accountable for progress toward these goals. To support this coordination function, HHS should establish a program management capability to direct and track the activities of internal and external stakeholders, and provide regular reports to ASPR, the Secretary of HHS, and the White House.

Recommendation 8-3. Public-Private Advisory Committee

HHS should establish a small advisory committee, comprised of representatives from the biotechnology, pharmaceutical and investment communities, to guide its engagement with industry.This committee's input should be considered seriously in all decisions and actions by the Department, given the importance of the relationship between the Federal Government and industry partners.

Recommendation 8-4. Oversight of Federal Investment in Influenza Vaccine Effort

HHS should also establish a dedicated entity, either within the Department (for example, under BARDA) or through an external organization, such as an FFRDC or PDP, to oversee the entire portfolio of Federal investments in the influenza vaccine enterprise. This entity should ensure that: (1) product development efforts proceed as expeditiously as possible, in full coordination with other activities supported by the US Government; (2) relevant government agencies (eg, FDA) have constant situational awareness of, and input to, these product development activities so issues can be identified and addressed as they arise; (3) companies have a channel for ongoing engagement with the US Government as data is gathered and product development proceeds; and (4) HHS has early awareness of external factors that could adversely impact companies' ability to advance product development efforts (eg, financial solvency, competing priorities, lack of critical expertise) and can raise these issues with company leadership before they jeopardize product development. Given the critical importance of these product development efforts for US preparedness, this kind of"hands on" engagement is necessary to ensure that these efforts proceed as expeditiously and predictably as possible.

This entity should track all elements of the product development effort, provide guidance to industry partners on regulatory and clinical development issues, identify problems and bottlenecks as they develop, bring them to the attention of the respective agency, and identify new technologies and potential partners for the Federal Government's influenza vaccine enterprise. It is essential that the entity have sufficient resources and staff with the necessary expertise in product development, commercialization, regulatory policy, portfolio management, financial planning and industrial relations.

Alignment with Broader Federal Medical Countermeasure Efforts

While these recommendations are driven by the recent H1 N1 pandemic, any reengineering of Federal Government's influenza vaccine efforts must be done in coordination with changes to the broader medical countermeasure

(MCM) enterprise. This should not be difficult—the attributes desired in the MCM enterprise are consistent with the approach proposed in this chapter. Moreover, influenza vaccines can serve as a timely and relevant pathfinder for changes to the United States Government's MCM strategy.

Specifically, the recommendations in this chapter are aligned with the Administration's prioritization of the following attributes in its MCM enterprise.

- The development of **multi-use platforms** and countermeasures is consistent with the recommendations to deploy platform technologies to speed up production of current influenza vaccines and to engineer next-generation influenza vaccines (Chapters 3, 4, and 5). These approaches will be relevant to both influenza and other public health threats, and the use of these technologies will help address both seasonal and pandemic influenza.
- **Partnerships and collaborations** are an essential element of the short, medium and long-term strategies proposed in this chapter.The development of partnerships and collaborations is most critical for industrial relations with the Federal government, given the pivotal role that the private sector will play in the achievement of these objectives.
- Regulatory innovation and advancement of **regulatory science,** particularly with regard to the mid and long-term approaches recommended here, are critically important to provide a roadmap for product development and certainty in the market for industry partners and the investment community.
- **Multidisciplinary project management capacity** must be established within the United States Government, possibly in concert with an external entity, to ensure that the complex interactions and partnerships are managed in a way that ensures the success of the enterprise.

Acknowledgments

PCAST wishes to express gratitude to the following individuals who contributed in various ways to the preparation of this chapter:

Joe Alper
Writer

Beth Bell
Associate Director for Science
National Center for Immunization and Respiratory Diseases
Centers for Disease Control and Prevention

Robert Coffman
Vice President and Chief Scientific Officer
Dynavax

Manon M. J. Cox
Chief Operating Officer
Protein Sciences

Nancy Cox
Influenza Division
Centers for Disease Control and Prevention

Bill Enright
President and Chief Executive Officer
Vaxi n Inc.

Anthony Fauci
Director, National Institute of Allergy and Infectious Diseases
National Institutes of Health

Michael Finney
Acting Chief Executive Officer
Vaxart

Bruce Gellin
Deputy Assistant Secretary for Health and Director
National Vaccine Program Office
Department of Health and Human Services

Douglas Given
Chief Executive Officer and Chairman

Vivaldi Blosciences

Jesse Goodman
Chief Scientist and Acting Deputy Commissioner
Food and Drug Administration

Richard Hatchett
Director for Medical Preparedness Policy
National Security Staff
Executive Office of the President

Doug Holtzman
Senior Program Officer
Bill and Melinda Gates Foundation

Bruce Innis
Vice President and Director
Global Clinical R&D, Vaccines for Influenza, MMR, Varicella and Dengue, GlaxoSmithKline

Paul E. Jarris
Executive Director
Association of State and Territorial Health Officials

Ti I Jolly
Associate Chief Medical Officer for Medical Readiness
Office of Health Affairs
Department of Homeland Security

George Kemble
Vice President, Vaccine Research and Development
Medimmune

Marie-Paule Kieny
Director, Initiative for Vaccine Research
World Health Organization

Richard Klausner
Managing Partner

The Column Group

James Lawler
Director for Medical Preparedness Policy
National Security Staff
Executive Office of the President

Nicole Lurie
Assistant Secretary for Preparedness and Response
Department of Health and Human Services

Frank Malinoski
Chief Medical Officer
Liquidia Technologies

Thomas Monath
Partner, Pandemic and Biodefense Fund
Kleiner Perkins Caufield & Byers

Thomas Muster
Chief Executive Officer and Chief Scientific Officer
AVIR Green Hills Biotechnology AG

Gary Nabel
Vaccine Research Center
National Institute of Allergy and Infectious Diseases
National Institutes of Health

Vasant Narasimhan
President, Vaccines & Diagnostics USA
Head, Vaccines North America
Novartis Vaccines and Diagnostics, Inc

Rino Rappuoli
Global Head of Vaccine Research
Novartis

Robin Robinson
Director

Biomedical Advanced Research & Development Authority (BARDA)

Alan Shaw
President & Chief Executive Officer
Vaxlnnate

Rahul Singhvi
President and Chief Executive Officer
Novavax

Tadataka Yamada
President
Global Health Program
Bill & Melinda Gates Foundation

APPENDIX A. LIST OF ACRONYMS

ASPR	Assistant Secretary for Preparedness and Response
BARDA	Biomedical Advanced Research and Development Authority
CDC	Centers for Disease Control and Prevention
DHS	Department of Homeland Security
DOD	Department of Defense
EOP	Executive Office of the President
FDA	Food and Drug Administration
FFRDC	Federally Funded Research and Development Center
HA	Hemagglutinin protein
HAI	Hemagglutinin inhibition
HBV	Hepatitis B
HHS	Department of Health and Human Services
HPV	Human papilloma virus
LAIV	Live attenuated influenza virus
M	Influenza virus matrix protein
MCM	Medical countermeasure
N	Neuraminidase protein
NIAID	National Institute of Allergy and Infectious Diseases
NIH	National Institutes of Health
NGIV	Next-generation influenza vaccine

PCAST	President's Council of Advisors on Science and Technology
PCR	Polymerase chain reaction
PDP	Product Development Partnership
TLR	Toll-like receptor
USDA	Department of Agriculture
VLP	Virus-like particle
WHO	World Health Organization

End Notes

1 President's Council of Advisors on Science and Technology. August 2009. *Report to the President on U.S. Preparations for 2009-H1N1 Influenza*. Available at www.whitehouse.gov/assets*_N1_Report.pdf.*

2 President's Council of Advisors on Science and Technology. August 2009. *Report to the President on U.S. Preparations for 2009-H1N1 Influenza*. Available at www.whitehouse.gov/assets

3 Obama BH."Remarks by the President in the State of the Union Addressf.lanuary 2010. Available at www.whitehouse.govithe-press-office/remarks-president-state-union-address.

4 The topical headings correspond to activities depicted on the time lines shown in Figure 2-1.

5 Robin Robinson, Director, Biomedical Advance Research and Development Authority, Personal Communication, June 9, 2010.

6 Matrajt L, Longini IM. Optimizing Vaccine Allocation at Different Points in Time during an Epidemic. *UW Biostatistics Working Paper Series* 2010, No. 363. Available at http://www.bepress.com/cgi/viewcontent.cgi?article=1202&context=uwbiostat.

7 Matrajt L, Longini IM. Optimizing Vaccine Allocation at Different Points in Time during an Epidemic. *UW Biostatistics Working Paper Series* 2010, No. 363. Available at http://www.bepress.com/cgi/viewcontent.cgi?article=1202&context=uwbiostat.

8 Williams TL, Luna L, et al. Quantification of Influenza Virus Hemagglutinins in Complex Mixtures using Isotope Dilution Tandem Mass Spectrometry. *Vaccine 2008*; 26:2510-20.

9 Department of Health and Human Services, Food and Drug Administration Center for Biologics Evaluation and Research. February 2010. *Guidance for Industry: Characterization and Qualification of Cell Substrates and Other Biological Materials Used in the Production of Viral Vaccines for Infectious Disease Indications*. Available at *http://www.fda.gov /downloads/BiologicsBloodVaccines/GuidanceComplianceRe%20* gulatoryInformation/GuidancesNaccines/UCM202439.pdf.

10 Belshe RB, Edwards KM, et al. Live Attenuated versus Inactivated Influenza Vaccine in Infants and Young Children. *New England Journal of Medicine* 2007; 356(7):685-696.

11 Ross TM, Mahmood K, et al. A Trivalent Virus-Like Particle Vaccine Elicits Protective Immune Responses against Seasonal Influenza Strains in Mice and Ferrets. *PLoS ONE 2009*; 4(6): e6032. Available at: *http://www.plosone.org/article/info:doi/10.1371/journal.pone.0006032.*

12 Perrone LA, Ahmad A, et al. Intranasal vaccination with 1918 influenza virus-like particles protects mice and ferrets from lethal 1918 and H5N1 influenza virus challenge. *Journal of Virology* 2009; 83(11):5726-34.

13 Streetlnsider. March 2010. Novavax (NVAX) *Announces Results for Influenza VLP Phase II* Available at: http://www.streetinsider.com/Corporate+News/Novavax+(NVAX)+Announces+Results+for+Influenza+VLP+Phase+11/ 5476269.html.

[14] Kwong P, Wilson I. HIV-1 and influenza antibodies: seeing antigens in new ways. *Nature Immunology* 2009; 10:573-578.

[15] Flanders Institute for Biotechnology. Universal Influenza Vaccine Tested Successfully In Humans. *ScienceDaily* 25 January 2008. Available at *www.sciencedaily.com/releases/2008/01/080124185522.htm.*

INDEX

C

G

H

K

L

M

N

O

P

V

W

Y

_influe